Essential psychiatry in general practice

D1355137

TL2879

Series Editors:
Manit Arya
Iqbal Shergill
Bob Mortimer

Other titles in the Essential General Practice Series include:
Essential Urology in General Practice

Note

Health and social care practice and knowledge are constantly changing and developing as new research and treatments, changes in procedures, drugs and equipment become available.

The authors, editor and publishers have, as far as is possible, taken care to confirm that the information complies with the latest standards of practice and legislation.

Essential Psychiatry in General Practice

Edited by

Afia Ali, Ian Hall and Andrew Dicker

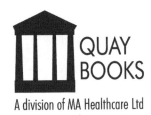

QUAY
BOOKS

A division of MA Healthcare Ltd

WM 100
R 2879

Quay Books Division, MA Healthcare Ltd, St Jude's Church, Dulwich Road, London
SE24 0PB

British Library Cataloguing-in-Publication Data
A catalogue record is available for this book

© MA Healthcare Limited 2010

ISBN-10: 1 85642 387 5
ISBN-13: 978 1 85642 387 8

Printed by CLE, Huntingdon, Cambridgeshire

Contents

Part 2
Legislation

Foreword

Although the Quality Outcome Framework (QOF) has biased attention towards physical medicine, much of the core of GP work remains mental and emotional health. At least a third of consultations are primarily for mental illness and this figure rises when the depression that often underlies unexplained physical symptoms and associated comorbidity is included. In almost all consultations, the emotional accompaniment of illness needs to be addressed. Consulting in primary care is a highly pressured and emotionally demanding activity.

As a practising GP, I would have had my copy of *Essential Psychiatry in General Practice* close to hand. Refreshingly, it takes a wide-angled view of psychiatry and includes chapters on medically unexplained symptoms, sexual disorders, women, children, learning disability, risk assessment and legislation – uses of the Mental Health Act as well as the ethics of consent. It is practical – lots of tables and lists of 'key points' – relevant, well researched, and written mainly by GPs and practising psychiatrists.

Whether or not to refer a patient to secondary services is a key decision in all primary care consultations, but it has additional complexity in mental health – the doctor's reaction to disturbed mental states may play a part; evidence of likely benefit may be unclear; subjective factors for the patient are of particular importance, and the question of stigma and the reluctance of the patient to be referred at all often arise. Thus the focus that the editors have chosen on the indications and appropriateness of referral to secondary care is likely to be particularly helpful for busy GPs in what is a highly complex subject.

Mental health services and treatments are proliferating. It is therefore all the more important for GPs and primary care mental health workers to have a reliable road map written by people familiar with the difficulties of the front line.

Andrew Elder FRCGP
President of the Balint Society
Consultant in General Practice and Primary Care
Marlborough Family Service
London NW8

Preface

A significant proportion of primary care consultations involve assessing and managing the mental health needs of patients. However, many General Practitioners (GPs) feel that they lack the skills and confidence in order to be able to diagnose and manage psychiatric conditions in primary care, particularly because of the lack of time available for consultations and issues related to managing risk.

This book is aimed at busy GPs and trainees and provides up-to-date, concise, practical guidelines on managing common mental health problems. This book will be essential to trainees sitting the MRCGP exams, but will also be useful to medical students, trainee doctors in related specialties and specialist nurses.

Most of the chapters have been written jointly by psychiatrists and GPs. Many of the authors are experts or have a special interest in their subject area, and the content of each chapter has been carefully selected and edited to ensure that it is relevant and accessible to GPs. Each chapter commences with case studies, followed by a discussion of relevant key points from the history, mental state examination and physical examination. The chapter is then followed by a discussion of relevant investigations and management options, including when it is necessary or appropriate to refer to secondary care. Each chapter is summarised by a list of key points at the end of the chapter.

We hope you find *Essential Psychiatry in General Practice* both a useful and enjoyable to read.

Series editors

Manit Arya MBChB, FRCS, FRCS(Urol)
Honorary CCT Fellow in Urology, King's College Hospital, London, UK

Iqbal S. Shergill BSc(Hons), MRCS(Eng), FRCS(Urol)
Consultant Urological Surgeon in Wrexham, North Wales, UK

Bob Mortimer FRCGP
General Practitioner in Swansea, South Wales, UK

The editors

Afia Ali MBBS, MRCPsych, MSc
Medical Research Council Clinical Research Fellow, Department of Mental Health Sciences, University College London

Ian Hall MA MB BChir MPhil FRCPsych
Consultant psychiatrist for people with intellectual disabilities at East London NHS Foundation Trust, Associate Program DirecStor for Specialty Training in Psychiatry of Learning Disability for the London Deanery, and Honorary Clinical Senior Lecturer in Psychiatry of Learning Disability at Queen Mary, University of London

Andrew Dicker MA MSc MBBS
General Practitioner in central London, Programme Director for the London Postgraduate Deanery at Royal Free Hospital Vocational Training Scheme for General Practice, and Honorary Senior Clinical Lecturer at Imperial College

Contributors

Mohamed Abdelghani MBBCh, MRCPsych
Specialty Registrar, Bexley Recovery Team, Oxleas NHS Foundation Trust

Afia Ali MBBS, MRCPsych, MSc
Medical Research Council Clinical Research Fellow, Department of Mental Health Sciences, University College London

Diana Andrea Barron MBBS MSc CPE MRCPsych
Clinical Research Fellow, Department of Mental Health Sciences, University College London

Jonathan Bickford
General Practitioner and GP Trainer, Oxford

Helen Bruce MBBS FRCPsych
Consultant Child and Adolescent Psychiatrist, Emanuel Miller Centre, East London NHS Foundation Trust and Honorary Clinical Senior Lecturer, Barts and the London School of Medicine and Dentistry

Marta Buszewicz MRCGP, MRCPsych
Senior Lecturer in Primary Care, Research Department of Primary Care & Population Health, University College London

Helen Caird BA, BSc, DClinPsych
Clinical Psychologist, Ridgeway Partnership NHS Trust

Lucy Carter MBBS, MRCGP
General Practitioner and Shared Care GP, City and Hackney Primary Care Trust

Vanessa Crawford MBBS, MRCPsych
Clinical Director, Specialist Addiction Service, East London NHS Foundation Trust

Andrew Crombie MRCPsych
Specialty Registrar, UCL Training Rotation, North London

Faye Dannhauser MA, MBBS, MRCP, MRCGP, DFFP
General Practitioner, Chigwell, Essex

Thomas Dannhauser MRCPsych
Consultant in Old Age Psychiatry, North Essex Partnership NHS Foundation Trust

Margaret Denman MB ChB, DFFP, MIPM
General Practitioner, Institute of Psychosexual Medicine, 12 Chandos Street, Cavendish Square, London

Andrew Dicker MBBS, MA MSc
General Practitioner and GP trainer, central London

Ian Hall MA, MB, BChir, MPhil, FRCPsych
Consultant Psychiatrist, East London NHS Foundation Trust

Michael Harding MB ChB Dip Obs (NZ) MRCGP
General Practitioner, London

Angela Hassiotis FRCPsych PhD
Senior Lecturer in the Psychiatry of Learning Disabilities, Department of Mental Health Sciences, University College London Medical School

Kazuya Iwata BSc, MBBS, MRCPsych, MSc
Specialty Registrar in General Adult Psychiatry, Camden and Islington NHS Foundation Trust

Benjamin Keene MBChB MRCPsych
Specialty Registrar in Liaison Psychiatry, Department of Psychological Medicine, Newham University Hospital, East London NHS Foundation Trust

Anthony Kerman MRCGP
General Practitioner, North London

Adrienne Key MB ChB MRCPsych
Member of Executive Committee Eating Disorder Section, Royal College of Psychiatrists and Lead Consultant at the Eating Disorder Service, Priory Hospital, Roehampton, South London

Michael Layton BSc MA MBBS MRCPsych PGDip (Forensic Mental Health)
Consultant Psychiatrist in Psychiatry of Learning Disability, Ridgeway Partnerships NHS Trust

Geoff Lawrence-Smith MBBS, MRCPsych
Consultant Psychiatrist, Bexley Recovery Team, Oxleas NHS Foundation Trust

Karl Marlowe MBChB, MSc, PgC-Ed, PgD-CBT, MRCPsych
Consultant Psychiatrist, East London NHS Foundation Trust, Burdett House, Mile End Hospital

Gary Marlowe
General Practitioner, De Beauvoir Surgery, North London

Shirlony Morgan MSc MRCPsych
Specialty Registrar in Old Age Psychiatry, London Deanery

Catherine Murgatroyd BSc, MbChB, MRCPsych
Locum Consultant in Perinatal Psychiatry, East London NHS Foundation Trust

Golda Mary Ninan MB.BCh., MRCGP, DRCOG, DFFP
General Practitioner, Chrisp Street Practice, 100 Chrisp Street, East London

Eleni Palazidou MD PhD MRCP FRCPsych
Consultant Psychiatrist, East London Foundation Trust

Jonathan Pimm MBBS, MSc, MRCPsych, MPhil, MD
Consultant in Primary Care Psychiatry and Honorary Senior Lecturer, East London NHS Foundation Trust and Queen Mary, University of London, Department of Psychiatry, Mile End Hospital

Adrian M. Raby MA MB BS BSc MRCGP
General Practitioner, Department of Primary Care and Social Medicine, Imperial College, London, Charing Cross Campus

Joanne Rodda MSc MRCPsych
Specialty Registrar in Old Age Psychiatry, London Deanery

Luke Solomons MBBS, MRCPsych, DGM
Consultant Psychiatrist in Old Age Psychiatry, Beechcroft CMHT for Older Adults, Hillcroft House, Rooke's Way, Thatcham

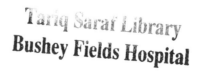

Joyce Solomons MBBS, MRCP, MS
Academic Clinical Fellow, Clinical Genetics, Churchill Hospital, Oxford Radcliffe NHS Trust, Oxford

Elza Tijo
Foundation Trainee in General Practice, Oxford

Ruth Townsend MbChB MRCGP DFFP
Salaried General Practitioner, Stepney Health Centre, Tower Hamlets PCT

Josephine Woolf MA BM BCh, MRCGP, MIPM
Institute of Psychosexual Medicine, 12 Chandos Street, Cavendish Square, London

PART I

Psychiatric disorders

CHAPTER 1

The psychiatric consultation

Jonathan Pimm and Golda Mary Ninan

Case history

A middle-aged woman with a long history of anxiety and depression who complained of low mood and occasional periods of elation was referred by her GP to a primary care psychiatrist. The patient was well presented and denied having any problems in her personal life. She was referred with a concern that she might be suffering from some form of manic depressive illness. A thorough history-taking over an hour revealed no abnormalities apart from three periods of 'elation'. Only when directly questioned about forensic problems did the patient break down in tears, explaining that she was facing a charge of shoplifting. Later, when her lawyer was contacted, it was found that the patient had a string of previous convictions for similar offences. At a subsequent consultation, the patient explained that she had never been 'so excited' as when she had managed to get out of a store without paying for clothes. On closer examination, it was clear that her elation followed her act of theft and that she was probably not suffering from a manic depressive disorder.

Introduction

Psychological ill health and psychiatric diseases rarely occur in isolation. Aetiological factors operate at all levels and in many cases are immediately obvious to the assessing physician. But in other cases, the causes of both patients' psychological and psychiatric disorders can be complicated and covert.

At the individual level, relationship difficulties, work-related problems or stressful neighbours are important common causal components of both psychological and psychiatric disorders seen in primary care. At the sociological level factors such as economic deprivation, unemployment, lack of education and ethnicity have been shown to be associated with most of the common psychiatric diseases. Both biological and genetic factors play a part in the causation of psychiatric and psychological conditions.

The degree to which different aetiological factors are responsible for causing a particular psychiatric or psychological disorder varies depending upon the individual, their environment and the disease. For example, some people develop depression or anxiety in stressful work environments, whereas others might thrive and indeed perform better in the same situation. With regard to conditions like schizophrenia and manic depression (also known as bipolar affective disorder), hereditary (genetic) factors are thought to be the major aetiological component.

Teasing out the importance of the various factors involved in the causation of both psychiatric and psychological disorders is vital to the understanding, management and treatment of such conditions.

Patients with both psychological and psychiatric problems often present with physical symptoms as indicators of their underlying distress or difficulties. The situation is often made more complicated when the presentation occurs at a time of crisis. Assessment of such individuals is difficult and often anxiety provoking – especially if the patient is unknown or unfamiliar to the attending physician.

In any consultation, the GP should endeavour to consider the presentation and its context. Both are important as they may provide information about the so-called 'illness narrative', or the story of the problem. Every patient has a narrative; it may appear superficial, trivial or even absent on first appraisal – but inevitably it is there somewhere. The purpose of the consultation is to try to find it, or at least help the patient to identify it, so that he or she may then begin to understand their difficulties and, if possible, begin to initiate change.

The more entrenched the patient's psychological problems, i.e. those starting early in the individual's life and continuing for several years, the less important the narrative. The reason for this is probably that the link between the original distress and the psychological difficulties which the patient continues to suffer has been lost; in essence the trauma and distress continue without a clear indication as to its source. Such patients – often labelled with the unhelpful term 'heartsink' – pose particular challenges in primary care.

Presentation

Patients' presentations of psychological problems are many and varied. However, the old adage that common things are common is as true in psychiatry as it is in any other specialty. The weird and wonderful diagnoses often named after eminent experts of days gone by are rare and probably best forgotten. Up to 40% of patients presenting to primary care have depression or a mixture of depression and anxiety. Many of these present with physical complaints as a manifestation of the psychological distress. Headaches, fatigue and poor sleep are among the problems most commonly faced by the primary care physician; rarely seen are nihilistic, delusional beliefs of rotting flesh or catatonic symptoms where the patient can be made to adopt various poses in a manner similar to an anglepoise lamp.

Once in the surgery, the ease with which a psychiatric diagnosis emerges is determined not only by the patient but also by the doctor. Research has found that patients often fear revealing feelings of unhappiness; they are sensitive to even the slightest cues from their doctors that might indicate lack of interest or impatience with such complaints.

Context

Knowledge of the context of the patient presenting to general practice with psychological complaints is in many respects more important than for patients seen in secondary care, since it is in hospital medicine that psychiatrists tend to deal with major disorders where the disease process is less influenced by the environment.

The idea that individuals at most times during their lives are asymptomatic is false; general surveys have found there is scarcely anyone who does not possess some psychological symptom or other. Further, the belief that the degree of seriousness of these symptoms is what motivates patients to seek help is also in many cases unfounded. Patients will delay seeking help for many reasons, including feeling guilty, ashamed, fearful, anxious or embarrassed, because of a dislike of their physician or because they have no one to care for their children while they go to the surgery. Even the phase of the Moon has been found to positively affect attendance in the primary care setting!

The patient's 'illness behaviour' – that is, the way a person behaves when they feel a need for better health – depends on many factors. Of particular relevance in psychiatric or psychological problems is their perception of their diseased status, cultural factors and stigma. The degree of fear of being given a psychiatric label will depend upon several factors, including the patient's past experience of services, knowledge of someone else's experience of the system or their treatment by the local community and beliefs about the treatments available (fear of side-effects and the development of dependency on drugs are of particular importance, specifically when considering adherence).

Conversely, many patients attend their GPs with seemingly minor difficulties. Their illness behaviour could be thought of as abnormal in certain circumstances. Sickness affords patients certain privileges, including the right to be exempted from normal activity (e.g. not going to work) and being regarded as in need of care and not being blamed for causing the illness (the sick role). However, the privileges also carry with them certain obligations, firstly in seeking medical advice and secondly not wanting to get well as quickly as possible. The doctor has an obligation to be objective and neutral (e.g. not to judge patients' behaviour on moral grounds) and to use his or her professional skills for the welfare of the patient and the community.

Overall, the severity of the patient's distress and his or her belief about the extent of the disability caused by the disease are the most important determinants of perceiving a need for care.

The impact of the individual doctor upon patients' consulting behaviours should not be underestimated. Some patients wait for several days before they can see a doctor of their choice. In many cases the original problem may have resolved by the time they get to see their physician; yet they may still decide to attend!

The Hungarian-born physician Michael Balint pioneered study of the interactions between doctors and their patients. In his classic text published in 1964, Balint remarked: 'The ability to listen is a new skill, necessitating a considerable though limited change in the doctor's personality' (Balint, 1964). Detailed recommendations as to how GPs should conduct consultations will not be given. For a comprehensive, and extremely readable, review on the general practice consultation the reader is advised to see Jill Thistlethwaite and Penny Morris's book (2006). Many different methods or models describing the process and structure of the consultation have been proposed over the past few decades – see Table 1.1.

The so-called 'patient-centred clinical method' is one that has been found the most suitable in the assessment and treatment of patients in primary care with both psychological and psychiatric complaints and details of this will be given later.

Preliminaries

The vexed problem of consultation length is one which has attracted much debate in primary care. Doctors continue to protest about a lack of time for the increasing number of tasks involved in routine consultations and they report greater satisfaction with surgeries if they only have to deal with simple patient agendas.

Table 1.1 A selection of different models of the consultation.

Byrne & Long (1976)	Stott and Davis (1979)	Pendleton et al. (1984)		Neighbour (1987)
(I) The doctor establishes a relationship with the patient	(I) Management of presenting problems	(I) To define the reason for the patient's attendance, including:	(1) the nature and history of the problems (2) their aetiology (3) the patient's ideas, concerns and expectations (4) the effects of the problems	Connecting
(II) The doctor either attempts to discover, or actually discovers the reason for the patient's attendance	(II) Management of continuing problems	(II) To consider other problems:	(i) continuing problems (ii) at-risk factors	Handing over
(III) The doctor conducts a verbal or physical examination, or both	(III) Modification of help-seeking behaviour	(III) With the patient, to choose an appropriate action for each problem		Summarising
(IV) The doctor, or the doctor and the patient together, or the patient alone consider(s) the condition	(IV) Opportunistic health promotion	(IV) To achieve a shared understanding of the problems with the patient		Safety-netting
(V) The doctor, and occasionally the patient details treatment or further investigation		(V) To involve the patient in the management and encourage him to accept appropriate responsibility		Housekeeping
(VI) The consultation is terminated – usually by the doctor		(VI) To use time and resources appropriately:	(i) in the consultation (ii) in the long term	
		(VII) To establish or maintain a relationship with the patient which helps to achieve the other tasks.		

The pressure of time and short consultation lengths – the UK average is 9.36 minutes – can increase the reluctance of doctors to engage with patients (Thistlethwaite and Morris, 2006). Patients themselves are acutely aware of time pressures in the surgery, and in particular people with depression have been found to be inhibited from fully disclosing their problems, thus preventing them making best use of the consultation. Doctors should be aware of patients' anxieties about time and allay these concerns by providing pre-emptive reassurance as a means of reinforcing their patient's sense of entitlement to consultation time.

Doctors with longer consultation times prescribe fewer drugs and offer more health promotion advice. They are also more likely to explore psychosocial problems.

Most modern surgeries are organised to allow the GP to maximise his or her time in the consultation room. Patients are 'arrived' on the computer screen when they present at the reception and, depending upon the sophistication of the practice, they will either be instructed by an electronic message board to go to a specific room and a specific doctor or they will be called by name, either by the GP or by a member of the receptionist team.

A handshake is a widely accepted introductory gesture. Clearly, consideration of the patient's age, cultural background and the doctor's prior knowledge of the patient may have a bearing on quite how widely accepted this is.

The position of the chairs within the consultation room probably does not make that much difference to the patient's feelings of security or comfort. The facilitative 45° angle favoured by examiners of the Royal College of Psychiatrists avoids confrontational eye contact and can help in putting the patient at ease – see Figure 1.1.

The dilemma of whether or not doctors should write anything down during interviews has largely been surpassed in general practice; most surgeries are paperless and some patients complain that the computer screen and keyboard have become the main focus of the GP's attention during the consultation.

Patients often rehearse what they plan to say to their doctors for many days before the appointment. They enter the surgery and begin with the so-called

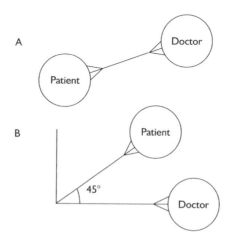

Figure 1.1 Different ways of looking at the patient: (a) the confrontational face-to-face approach and (b) the facilitative 45° angle approach.

'opening gambit' statement; this is sometimes preceded by a more spontaneous remark known as the 'curtain raiser'. The opening gambit provides the GP with the overt agenda.

An uninterrupted patient will usually conclude this initial monologue within 30 seconds but doctors commonly interject before this time. This only results in shortening the gambit by about 10 seconds. Thus it is recommended the patient be given a little free rein (within reason!) to speak without interruption at the start of any consultation.

Attention needs to be maintained right to the end of the interview so as not to miss the so-called 'doorknob comment', which (as its name suggests) is made just as the patient is about to leave the room.

The patient-centred approach

The improvement of doctors' communication skills and the use of a patient-centred approach in general practice are likely to be the most important factors that will lead to better management of mental health problems.

The patient-centred method aims to cover the following six main areas:

1. The patient's experience and expectations regarding the disease
2. An understanding of the patient as a whole person rather than just a symptom
3. The seeking of common ground regarding management
4. Health promotion
5. An enhancement of the doctor–patient relationship

and

6. To be realistic in its achievements given limitations of time

The patient-centred approach has been extensively researched and repeatedly found to show many benefits and advantages over other models of consultation – particularly the doctor-centred one. Patient concordance with medication has been shown to be higher, disease outcomes have been demonstrated to be improved and a decrease in rates of malpractice claims has also been confirmed.

When questioned about the various facets of their consultations, patients identified communication, partnership and health promotion as being the most important to them. About 60% of patients expressed the desire for an examination, and only a quarter wanted a prescription (Little *et al.*, 2001).

However, it is probably fair to say that 'one size does not fit all' with regard to adopting all facets of the patient-centred consultation approach. In reality it is necessary to adopt a more flexible approach to the model, taking into account the patient's desire for information or for sharing in the decision-making process, for example.

GP trainees often use the acronym ICE and E as a checklist of items to cover during the consultation. I = ideas (beliefs of the patient regarding cause of the problem or problems), C = concerns (worries about the problem or problems), E = expectations (the expectations the patient has regarding the problem or problems) and E = effects (how the problem or problems affect the patient's life).

Each patient should be approached without preconceived ideas. It should be appreciated that often, unless directly asked, the patient may not volunteer important information (Barry *et al.*, 2000). Personal details involving sexual activities, the use of drugs and alcohol, suicidal ideas and financial or legal problems are clearly sensitive subjects. But often, unless the question is posed, such information may not be volunteered spontaneously. More importantly, without knowing such information, the GP will never be able to offer the appropriate treatment or help.

Patients do not usually take offence, provided questions are put sensitively. Specifically, with regard to self-harm or suicide, research provides ample evidence to reassure the GP reluctant to ask about such matters that questioning the patient will not affect the likelihood of them killing themselves.

It has been shown that doctors report greater satisfaction with consultations if they only have to deal with simple patient agendas. Further, a lack of confidence has been associated with GPs being reluctant to tackle all the complexities of their patients' problems. It has also been shown that doctors may be overwhelmed by the scope and nature of their patients' troubles – even if they are able and willing to explore ideas, concerns and expectations in full. Doctors may also feel powerless in the face of certain patient expectations (Thistlethwaite and Morris, 2006).

The establishment of a trusting rapport with the patient is without doubt an important task of any consultation; this may take time and ideally requires several appointments. However, in today's general practices, doctors may not be afforded such a luxury because not only do patients move regularly, but GPs are often employed on temporary contracts and in surgeries with multiple partners. Repeated attenders may have to see a different physician on each occasion they seek help.

Difficult and demanding circumstances

Many consultations in general practice can be challenging, difficult and demanding. Such circumstances may arise when, for example, the patient com-

plains of numerous physical problems for which there is no obvious pathological cause, or the patient is chronically depressed and no medication or psychological therapy has made any difference. There is no simple solution to such
situations. Recommendations on how to adopt a calm, empathetic approach or
even the use of a double-appointment slot to see the patient are not particularly
helpful to the jobbing GP in a busy practice.

It is worth appreciating that patients affect their doctors; people with complaints of unhappiness and recurring, incurable, physical aches and pains are
particularly troublesome to the psyche of the physician. Derogatory classifications and descriptions have been given to patients who produce such strong
feelings in doctors. The use of such terms is unhelpful and does not aid the
doctor–patient relationship, nor does it aid any management or treatment
programme. Such patients tend to be remembered and thought of as frequent
attenders.

Dealing with such patients brings despair; empathy is often lost, and anger
and frustration develop. The need for the GP to understand his or her disem-
powerment is a necessary starting point for the possibility of helping such
patients. These feelings do not need to be communicated to the patient, but a
realisation on the part of the physician is sufficient. A more complete understanding of the patient's story begins to put the humanity back into the situation. The patient no longer becomes a long list of entries on the computer
screen but someone with real problems and concerns.

Discovering the patient's story may restore the doctor's empathy, and
although it may not offer management solutions, such knowledge should
improve the doctor–patient relationship (Thistlethwaite and Morris, 2006).
GPs often reflect upon the reasons why such patients repeatedly come and
see them when there is no obvious improvement in the individual's condition.
The importance of the interaction is sometimes revealed when the doctor is no
longer available for a prolonged period of time, e.g. maternity or sick leave.
Patients will often confess that their consultations with the now absent doctor
were an absolute life-saver. Further, it is important to appreciate that for some
patients the only meaningful conversation they have is with a health professional. The surgery is a point of social contact for isolated and lonely people
without family support (Thistlethwaite and Morris, 2006). It may be a cliché to
say that the interaction is itself therapeutic – but frequently this is the feedback
obtained when a particular GP is no longer available.

Out of all so-called repeat attenders in primary care, approximately 60%
complain of depressive symptoms (Dowrick *et al.*, 2000). Clearly then, they
make up a large proportion of primary care work if one appreciates that only
5% of patients account for about 20% of all consultations (Neal *et al.*, 1998).
Patients complaining of so-called medically unexplained symptoms (also
known as chronic multiple functional somatic symptoms or CMFSs) make
up another large faction of frequent attenders in primary care (see Chapter 7).

Psychological factors have been clearly found to be involved in the generation of these symptoms in approximately 60% of cases. Experts have repeatedly argued for the adoption of a chronic disease management approach to such patients. Other chronic conditions, such as diabetes and coronary heart disease, are treated with such a model which involves building close links with community resources, support for self-management by patients and consultancy from specialist colleagues. Using a chronic disease management approach for patients suffering with long-term depression and conditions where continued underlying psychological distress plays a major part in perpetuating the distress may not be possible – particularly in the current climate of austerity – since it would require additional funding. However, the following points adapted from Bass and May (2002) are worth bearing in mind:

1. Arrange regular appointments to see the patient. Such a strategy sends a clear message to the frequent attendee that the GP continues to be concerned and that his or her problems are being taken seriously. Furthermore, it may set a boundary on the patient's attending behaviour.
2. Consultations should be used to focus upon things that the patient 'can do' rather than those things he or she 'cannot do'.
3. The GP should look to containment of the problem rather than trying to cure the complaint or complaints.
4. The GP should try to minimise the patient's contacts with other specialists or practitioners. However, in order to give the particular GP a 'break' it might be appropriate that a practice partner or colleague offer a second opinion or take over the case for a while.
5. Regular discussion of the case with colleagues or other practice staff can also help.
6. The consultation should not be used to focus upon the patient's problem or problems unless of course there is a change in symptoms or complaints.
7. Simple reinforcement of the message that by focusing upon the symptoms the patient will set up a vicious circle whereby the more he or she thinks about the problem the greater the problem will be.

Finally, the despairing doctor may be helped by appreciating that only one third of frequent consulters continue using resources in an excessive manner after 12 months have elapsed. In essence, something changes in two thirds of frequent attenders that stops them consulting their GP; what changes may be difficult to discern in many cases, but could include things like the passage of the crisis when a relationship problem resolves; the patient feels the GP is not really any good for their particular difficulty; or maybe an unexpected event happens. Maybe the patient gets the job they had been repeatedly applying for or maybe he or she falls in love or even wins the Lottery!

Key points

- Psychiatric illness must be seen in the context of the patient's psychological, sociological and biological makeup.
- Patients commonly present with physical complaints when they are suffering from psychological or psychiatric disorders.
- Many models and methods have been used and described over the past twenty years to understand and aid consultation practices in primary care.
- The patient-centred approach is one method that has been widely adopted by GPs.
- Patients should be approached without preconceived ideas. Unless directly asked, they may not volunteer important information necessary to make the correct diagnosis.

Further reading and bibliography

Balint, M. (1964) *The Doctor, His Patient and the Illness.* Pitman Medical, London.

Barry, C. A., Bradley, C. P., Britten, N., Stevenson, F. A. and Barber, N. (2000) Patients' unvoiced agendas in general practice consultations: qualitative study. *British Medical Journal*, **320**, 1246–50.

Bass, C. and May, S. (2002) Chronic multiple functional somatic symptoms. *British Medical Journal*, **325**, 323–6.

Dowrick, C. F., Bellon, J. A. and Gomez, M. J. (2000) GP frequent attendance in Liverpool and Granada: the impact of depressive symptoms. *British Journal of General Practice*, **50**, 361–5.

Little, P., Everitt, H., Williamson, I., Warner, G., Moore, M., Gould, C., Ferrier K. and Payne, S. (2001) Preferences of patients for patient centred approach to consultation in primary care: observational study. *British Medical Journal*, **322**, 468–72.

Neal, R. D., Heywood, P. L., Morley, S., Clayden, A. D. and Dowell, A. C. (1998) Frequency of patients' consulting in general practice and workload generated by frequent attenders: comparisons between practices. *British Journal of General Practice*, **48**, 895–8.

Thistlethwaite, J. and Morris, P. (2006) *The Patient–Doctor Consultation in Primary Care – Theory and Practice.* Royal College of General Practitioners, London.

CHAPTER 2

Depression and other common mental disorders

Jonathan Pimm and Golda Mary Ninan

Case study

The patient was aged 24 years and had been attending her GP's surgery for several months complaining of unhappiness. She also reported spending a great deal of time washing. She said she was taking about five baths every day because she felt dirty. According to her mother, she had to wash the kitchen three or four times a day because it was 'contaminated with germs'.

The GP was concerned that the patient was suffering from obsessive compulsive disorder and wanted her to be seen by a psychiatrist. On examination, it was found that the patient's home was inhabited by three large dogs which were allowed to wander freely all over the house; they were essentially under the supervision of the patient's mother who took little notice of their state of hygiene. The animals left hair on the patient's bed and jumped up onto the worktops in the kitchen.

The patient's story became more complicated when she stated that she had been depressed since she was about 15 years of age; the time when she began experimenting with ecstasy and cocaine. Her mood had taken a further downturn in recent months after a previously violent partner had returned to the neighbourhood having obtained early release from a 10 year prison sentence. He had been found guilty of a vicious attack on a family member soon after attacking the patient.

Introduction

The grumble of unhappiness in a busy afternoon surgery can be one of the most difficult complaints GPs have to deal with. It is certainly one of the most common. The situation can be especially frustrating because patients with sadness at the core of their presentation often keep coming back time and again.

Misery, sadness or unhappiness are found in the context of many diseases. It may be one of a combination of symptoms appearing in a physical disease – for example in hypothyroidism or Cushing's disease. It may also be seen in the context of drug and alcohol misuse. In the vast majority of cases it is seen in patients suffering from both psychological and psychiatric disorders. By far the most common psychiatric diseases, where unhappiness or low mood is the core symptom, are those of depression or a mixture of depression and anxiety (known as mixed anxiety and depressive disorder).

Depression and mixed anxiety and depressive disorder (MADD) make up most of the cases of psychological and psychiatric diseases seen in primary care. The remaining cases are made up of obsessive compulsive disorder, panic disorder and phobias – see Figure 2.1. It must be stressed that, in reality, many cases seen in general practice have symptoms of several different disorders, as illustrated in the case study above.

GPs have repeatedly been criticised for failing to recognise patients suffering from depression. Previously, research found that up to 50% of all cases of depression presenting to primary care were not picked up. Recently, however, the situation has been found to be a little more complex; cases are not simply recognised or un-recognised. In reality, the ability of the doctor to diagnose the disease varies depending upon the severity of the symptoms. Patients with

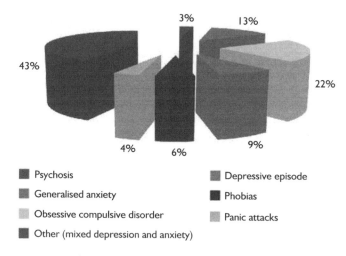

Figure 2.1 The prevalence of psychiatric disease.

more severe symptoms are almost always diagnosed by GPs. Further, it has been found that even when a case is missed initially, it is usually picked up at subsequent visits. In reality, the rather condemning figure of one in two cases being missed is more like one in seven.

The problem of under-diagnosis is compounded by the fact that many depressed or anxious patients present to their family doctors complaining of somatic symptoms. In addition, many patients in primary care diagnosed with medically unexplained symptoms have been found to be suffering from depression, MADD or some other form of psychological problem, e.g. a somatoform disorder.

As well as under-diagnosis, it has been reported that GPs under-treat patients complaining of depression and other common mental disorders (CMDs). The reasons for this under-treatment include beliefs that the medication is ineffective and concerns that patients will not take antidepressants even if they are offered.

The difficulties of under-diagnosis and under-treatment are also tied up with the contentious issue of how to clearly distinguish depression and the other common mental disorders from normal unhappiness and worry.

Before turning to the conditions individually, the term *neurosis* will be discussed in an attempt to illustrate how each of the separate disorders became recognised.

Neurosis

Neurosis, or neurotic disorders, lies on the psychiatric illness spectrum between psychotic conditions and normal mental health. The term *neurosis* was first used to mean any disorder of the nervous system without any obvious symptoms or signs of physical disease. Freud believed the neuroses were mainly the result of the discharge of damned up instinctual drives, e.g. sexual energy (or libido).

The division into specific diagnoses came with the discovery of antidepressant drugs. The tricyclic antidepressant imipramine was claimed to be effective in treating spontaneous panic attacks and resulted in the classifications of panic disorder (PD) with or without agoraphobia. Benzodiazepines were reported to be useful in the treatment of generalised anxiety, but much less effective in the treatment of panic attacks. The condition of generalised anxiety disorder (GAD) was conceived as an illness better treated with benzodiazepines. The specificity of treatments for the different conditions has failed to stand the test of time although classification of the disorders remains unaltered.

Aetiology

Current understanding of the causes of neurotic disorders is based on knowledge derived from the three main groupings of aetiology of all psychiatric disease – biological, psychological and social. Under the biological umbrella, genes have been found to make a contribution. The neurological mechanisms underpinning such genetic susceptibilities have mainly been elucidated through scientific investigation of the medications used to treat the disorders; these are the $GABA_A$ benzodiazepine receptor complex, the 5-HT1_A and 5-HT2_C receptors and the noradrenergic group.

Psychological appreciation of the mechanisms behind the development of anxiety disorders comes from behaviourists' studies. Phobias, for example, result from the association of neutral stimuli with fear-evoking events.

Social factors are clearly important in understanding the cause of neurotic conditions; there is a strong association with problems such as isolation, lack of support, unemployment and poverty.

Depression

Introduction

The number of patients suffering from depression in general practice is high; by 2020 depression will rank second only to cardiovascular disease as a global cause of disability. Some researchers believe depression may occur in as many as 51.5% of people attending their general practice (Kessler *et al.*, 1999). Other investigators have made more conservative estimates of approximately a quarter of patients in primary care. Whichever figure is correct, the problem is mainly handled by GPs in primary care and therefore must be one a family doctor is capable of dealing with; only about 10% of all psychiatric morbidity reaches the level of secondary care and a psychiatrist.

Aetiology

Stressful life events, including low income and financial strain, unemployment, problems at work, social isolation and poor housing have been found to be potent predictors of depression.

A previous history of depression, gender, age, genetics and personality style are some of the independent risk factors known to contribute to the development of depression.

Certain personality characteristics have been found to predict which patients become depressed. For example, individuals dependent upon interpersonal relationships and concerned about disapproval by others have been found to be susceptible to depression after negative interpersonal events such as the death of a loved one.

Historical perspective

Numerous strategies have been devised over the past 20 years in an attempt to overcome the problems of diagnosing and treating depression and the other CMDs. Educational training, treatment guidelines, financially incentivised questionnaire-led diagnostic programmes and publicity awareness campaigns have all been shown to be ineffective despite initial optimism.

The latest thinking is that depression and the other CMDs should ideally be managed in the same way as diseases like diabetes or rheumatoid arthritis. Such a method (known as the chronic care model) of treatment would involve multidisciplinary teams intensively case-managing patients throughout the whole of their illness. Such a model would have significant opportunity costs.

Until resources become available so that the chronic care model can be universally adopted, the only clear recommendation for doctors dealing with depression and the other CMDs is that they endeavour to undertake a comprehensive history and assessment.

Assessment

A psychiatrist working in a hospital or outpatient clinic usually has an hour or more to assess new patients; for the doctor in primary care this is an enviable luxury. In most cases however, the diagnosis becomes apparent after several short consultations undertaken over a period of days or weeks. The appropriate course of action can then be taken by the practitioner armed with a full understanding of what he is dealing with.

Mood and affect

Before looking at the current diagnostic criteria for depression and the other CMDs it is worth considering the symptom of unhappiness in a little more detail.

Psychiatrists talk about a patient's mood rather than his or her sadness. They also describe the patient's affect. Affect, according to psychiatrists, is like the weather, whereas mood is like the climate. Mood should be thought of as an emotional state quantifying happiness or unhappiness present over the longer term. In a sense, it is the pervasive feeling the patient experiences most of the time.

Mood should not be thought of as the minute to minute, hour to hour change in the happiness or unhappiness state. This state is experienced by all humans. It changes rapidly and this is labelled by psychiatrists as the patient's affect. Further, the patient's affect can and often does alter during the course of the consultation – one moment there are tears and sadness, the next there are giggles and smiles. Alternatively, the patient's affect may be flattened and unreactive such that all their spark or zest for life has been swamped by their misery.

Further indications as to the nature of the condition can be obtained by enquiring about the duration of the symptoms. The length of suffering often gives a pointer as to how risky the patient's state is. Unhappiness of a couple of days may be best left alone: unhappiness of years could probably do with a few more consultations and a little more questioning focusing on past experiences and past contact with psychiatric services.

Risk assessment

Every patient found to be suffering from depression and other CMDs should be questioned about suicidal ideas and plans. Such enquiry generates no additional risk to the patient, so there should be no hesitation in asking about the subject.

The matter may be introduced in a variety of ways, and the GP should adopt one that he or she is comfortable with and stick with it. An assessment of ideas of suicide may be made by simply asking the patient whether he or she has ever felt that life was not worth living. The question should be followed up by enquiry about any plans or thoughts on how the patient would end his or her life.

Finally, the patient should be asked about previous episodes of self-harm and self-poisoning. A record of the number of times the patient has self-harmed and self-poisoned, the circumstances surrounding the event and the actions which followed should all be documented.

Diagnosis

The screening questions of the Patient Health Questionnaire – 2 (PHQ-2) have been shown to be sensitive and specific – see Figure 2.2. These are:

PHQ-2

Over the past two weeks, how often have you been bothered by any of the following problems?

Little interest or pleasure in doing things.
0 = Not at all
1 = Several days
2 = More than half the days
3 = Nearly every day

Feeling down, depressed, or hopeless.
0 = Not at all
1 = Several days
2 = More than half the days
3 = Nearly every day

Total point score: _____

Figure 2.2 Patient Health Questionnaire 2 – PHQ-2.

1. Over the last two weeks, how often have you been bothered by little interest or pleasure in doing things?
2. Over the last two weeks, how often have you been feeling down, depressed or hopeless?

Answering anything other than 'Not at all' to either of the questions can be considered a positive test result and should prompt further examination. For the more diligent GP, scores of above 3 on the PHQ-2 have been shown to be sensitive and specific for picking up cases of depression.

The Patient Health Questionnaire – 9 (PHQ-9) has become the most widely used instrument for GPs suspecting a depressive disorder. This is an easy to use questionnaire which the patient fills in. It scores each of the nine criteria for depression found in the American diagnostic system, the DSM-IV (*Diagnostic and Statistical Manual of Mental Disorders*, 4th edition)) as '0' (not at all), '1' (on several days), '2' (more than half the days), '3' (nearly every day) depending on whether the patient has been 'bothered' by a list of nine problems over the previous two weeks – see Figure 2.3.

The questionnaire's validity has been assessed against an independent structured mental health professional interview. A PHQ-9 score of greater than or equal to 10 has a sensitivity of 88% and specificity of 88% for major depression. A score on the PHQ-9 of 0–4 represents no disease, 10–14 moderate depression, 15–19 moderately severe depression and 20–27 severe disease.

The ICD-10 classification of disease is the diagnostic system mainly used by psychiatrists in the UK.

PATIENT HEALTH QUESTIONNAIRE (PHQ-9)

NAME: _____   DATE:_____

Over the *last 2 weeks*, how often have you been bothered by any of the following problems? (use "✓" to indicate your answer)	Not at all	Several days	More than half the days	Nearly every day
1. Little interest or pleasure in doing things	0	1	2	3
2. Feeling down, depressed, or hopeless	0	1	2	3
3. Trouble falling or staying asleep, or sleeping too much	0	1	2	3
4. Feeling tired or having little energy	0	1	2	3
5. Poor appetite or overeating	0	1	2	3
6. Feeling bad about yourself—or that you are a failure or have let yourself or your family down	0	1	2	3
7. Trouble concentrating on things, such as reading the newspaper or watching television	0	1	2	3
8. Moving or speaking so slowly that other people could have noticed. Or the opposite—being so fidgety or restless that you have been moving around a lot more than usual	0	1	2	3
9. Thoughts that you would be better off dead, or of hurting yourself in some way	0	1	2	3

add columns: [_____] + [_____] + [_____]

(Healthcare professional: For interpretation of TOTAL,   **TOTAL:** [_____]
please refer to accompanying scoring card.)

Figure 2.3 Patient Health Questionnaire 9 – PHQ-9.

ICD-10 Diagnostic criteria for depression – mild, moderate, severe

There is some overlap between the ICD-10 criteria and the PHQ-9, but the ICD-10 allows the physician to categorise the patient more specifically. The initial classification in the manual describes three varieties – namely mild (F32.0), moderate (F32.1) and severe (F32.2 and F32.3).

The manual lists core, other and somatic symptoms (see Table 2.1). For the three grades of severity (mild, moderate and severe), a duration of at least two weeks is usually required for diagnosis.

Table 2.1 ICD-10 Diagnostic criteria for depression.

Core symptoms	Other symptoms	Somatic symptoms*
Depressed mood	Reduced concentration and attention	Loss of interest or pleasure in activities that are normally enjoyable
Loss of interest and enjoyment (also known as anhedonia)	Reduced self-esteem and self-confidence	Lack of emotional reactivity to normally pleasurable surroundings and events
Reduced energy leading to increased fatigability and diminished activity	Ideas of guilt and unworthiness (even in a mild type of episode)	Waking in the morning 2 hours or more before the usual time
	Bleak and pessimistic views of the future	Depression worse in the morning
	Ideas or acts of self-harm or suicide	Objective evidence of definite psychomotor retardation or agitation (remarked on or reported by other people)
	Diminished sleep	Marked loss of appetite
	Diminished appetite	Weight loss (often defined as 5% or more of body weight in the past month)
		Marked loss of libido

*The somatic **syndrome** is defined as being present only when at least four of the above somatic symptoms are definitely present.

Mild depression

Mild depression is defined by the presence of at least two of the core symptoms (listed in Table 2.1) being present with at least two of the others (Table 2.1) for at least two weeks. An individual with a mild depressive episode is usually distressed by the symptoms and has some difficulty in continuing with ordinary work and social activities, but will probably not cease to function completely.

Mild depression is classified further with regard to the presence or absence of the somatic syndrome (note again: for this to be present, four of the somatic symptoms need to be present).

Moderate depression

Moderate depression is defined by the presence of at least two of the core symptoms being present with at least three (preferably four) of the other symptoms for at least two weeks.

Moderate depression is classified further with regard to the presence or absence of the somatic syndrome.

Severe depression

This is defined by the presence of all three of the core symptoms with at least four of the other symptoms, some of which should be of severe intensity. In a severe depressive episode the sufferers usually show considerable distress or agitation, unless retardation is a marked feature. Loss of self-esteem or feelings of uselessness or guilt are likely to be prominent and suicide is a distinct danger. It is presumed that the somatic syndrome is almost always present in a severe depressive episode.

Severe depression is classified further with regard to the presence or absence of psychotic symptoms. If delusions, hallucinations or a depressive stupor are present, then the patient should be thought of as psychotic.

Other types of depression

Recurrent depressive disorder

The ICD-10 classification describes a recurrent depressive disorder as being characterised by repeated episodes of illness of a mild, moderate or severe degree without any history of independent mood elevation and over activity that might fulfil the criteria of mania.

The episodes last between three and 12 months (median duration about six months) and recovery is usually complete before the next episode begins again. Individual episodes of any severity are often precipitated by stressful life events. The disorder is about twice as common in women as in men.

The treatment of recurrent depressive disorder will be considered separately below.

Dysthymia

The ICD-10 classification lists dysthymia as a chronic lowering of mood which fails to fulfil the criteria for recurrent depressive disorder of either a mild or moderate severity. Sufferers of dysthymia usually have periods of days or weeks when they describe themselves as well. But most of the time (often months at a time) they feel tired and depressed. Everything is an effort and nothing is enjoyed. They brood and complain. They sleep badly and feel inadequate – but they are usually able to cope with the basic demands of everyday life.

Some of these patients were previously labelled as 'depressive personality disorder'.

Anxiety disorders

Here the two disorders with anxiety as a core feature – generalised anxiety disorder and mixed anxiety and depressive disorder – will be described and discussed. However, the division between the two is rather artificial and certainly diagnostically unclear.

Anxiety – classified as generalised anxiety disorder

The essential feature is anxiety which is generalised and persistent and 'free-floating' – that is, not restricted to or predominating in a particular situation or environment. The symptoms should have the following elements:

1. Apprehension (worries about future misfortunes, feeling 'on edge', difficulty in concentrating
2. Increased motor tension (restless fidgeting, tension headaches, trembling, inability to relax)
3. Increased autonomic nervous system activity leading to a variety of symptoms including sweating, light-headedness, tachycardia, tachypnoea, epigastric discomfort, dizziness, dry mouth and palpitations

These symptoms must be present on most days for at least several weeks at a time and usually for several months. About 1–5% of the general population report having generalised anxiety disorder. Most people with generalised anxiety disorder also have other mood or anxiety disorders.

Mixed anxiety and depression

The mixture of anxiety and depressive symptoms in primary care patients has led to much debate and research. Considering epidemiological surveys have found it to be the most common presentation in general practice, it seems bizarre that it is regarded in the ICD-10, as a 'sub-syndromal' disorder. The diagnosis is allowed only if neither the anxiety nor the depressive symptoms reach the threshold for either disorder. The dislike of diagnosis may have something to do with its acronym (MADD – mixed anxiety and depressive disorder).

Other neurotic conditions

The other neurotic conditions, including obsessive compulsive disorder, specific phobias and adjustment disorders, will not be discussed here. Only panic disorder and agoraphobia will be mentioned because they appear in the treatment guidelines from the National Institute for Health and Clinical Excellence (NICE, 2004) under the general heading of anxiety.

Panic disorder and agoraphobia

The diagnosis of panic disorder was introduced in 1980 in the USA largely because of evidence that tricyclic antidepressants specifically blocked panic attacks. The disorder is characterised by two components: recurrent panic attacks and anticipatory anxiety. The essential feature of the recurrent attacks of severe anxiety (panic) is that they are not restricted to any particular situation or set of circumstances and are therefore unpredictable. During the period of panic the patient may experience several different symptoms including:

- palpitations
- sweating
- trembling or shaking
- sensations of shortness of breath or being smothered
- sensation of choking
- chest pain or discomfort
- nausea or abdominal discomfort
- feeling dizzy, unsteady, light headed or faint
- derealisation (feelings of unreality) or depersonalisation (being detached from oneself)
- fear of losing control or going crazy
- fear of dying
- paraesthesia
- chills or hot flushes

The anticipatory anxiety is an intense fear of having another panic attack, which continues on throughout the periods between the actual attacks. Some patients go on to develop agoraphobia (see below for details) in association with the panic attacks; in this case the disorder is known as panic disorder with agoraphobia.

Panic disorder is associated with depression and other anxiety disorders. About a third of patients with depression present with panic disorder. Throughout their lives about half of patients with panic disorder will develop depression and about half of depressed patients will develop panic disorder. Large population surveys have found that clearly defined panic attacks occur in approximately 10% of the population.

Agoraphobia is basically an anxiety about being in places or situations from which escape is difficult (or embarrassing) or in which help may not be available. Again the symptoms produced by the anxiety are the same as those listed above in the discussion about generalised anxiety disorder. Agoraphobia also commonly occurs in association with other neurotic conditions – particularly depression and panic disorder.

Physical causes of depression and anxiety

In all patients presenting with depression and a mixture of depression and anxiety symptoms, it is necessary to exclude any physical cause. Some of the more common physical causes which need to be borne in mind are:

- Endocrine disorders – hypo- and hyperthyroidism, hypoglycaemia, hypo- and hypercalcaemia (and rarely seen but commonly remembered) – phaeo-chromocytoma.
- Cardiac disorders – hypoxia, angina, arrhythmias, congestive heart failure, mitral valve prolapse
- Pulmonary disorders – hypoxia, chronic obstructive pulmonary disease, pneumonia, hyperventilation, pulmonary embolism
- Neurological disorders – partial complex seizures, encephalitis, post-concussion syndrome, sleep disorders
- Metabolic disorders – vitamin B12 deficiency, porphyria
- Stimulant toxicity – caffeine, sympathomimetic medications or drugs (cocaine, crack, amphetamines)
- Withdrawal syndromes – alcohol, benzodiazepines, barbiturates, opiates, etc.
- Delirium of any aetiology – or acute confusional syndrome

Management

Guidelines on how to treat anxiety and depression have been produced by NICE (2004 and 2009 respectively).

The treatment recommendations for depression are based upon clinical ICD-10 diagnoses and adopt a so-called 'stepped care' approach – see Table 2.2. The treatments for depression fall into four main categories:

1. Watchful waiting – essentially observation
2. Self-help treatments – which can either be done by the patient alone or guided by a primary care mental health worker
3. Psychological treatments – these are in two main categories; in essence short or long term
4. Medication

The basis of treatment protocols requires an accurate diagnosis. Once the problem is clear then the appropriate treatment can be prescribed. This can be simply summarised as:

- Mild depression – watchfully waiting with or without self-help, computerised psychological therapy or brief psychological interventions
- Moderate depression – antidepressant and psychological (talking) therapy
- Severe depression – complex psychological interventions and antidepressant or other medications and ECT

The treatment options for anxiety (including generalised anxiety disorder and panic disorder with or without agoraphobia) as outlined in the NICE guidelines (2004) are essentially, antidepressants, self-help, guided self-help and psychological treatments. These options will be considered in more detail below. The only other major point to note in the NICE guidelines for anxiety disorders is that drugs like benzodiazepines and other anxiolytics are not recommended (2004).

Antidepressants and other psychopharmacological treatments

Antidepressants (see Chapter 17 for more details)

The general rule with regard to treatment of depression and the other CMDs is to start with a serotonin reuptake inhibitor (e.g. citalopram, sertraline, fluox-

Table 2.2 The stepped care model for depression (NICE guidelines 2009).

Step	Service provider	Role	Treatment/management
One	GP, practice nurse	Recognition/identification of depressive episode	Assessment
Two	GP, primary care mental health worker	Mild depression	Watchful waiting, self-help resources, computerised CBT, sleep hygiene, brief psychological interventions
Three	GP, primary care mental health worker	Moderate to severe depression	Antidepressant, social support, psychological therapy
Four	Community mental health teams, crisis resolution/home treatment teams	Severe depression – treatment resistant, psychotic depression, recurrent depressive disorder	Antidepressant, combined treatments, psychological interventions
Five	Inpatient care, crisis resolution/home treatment teams	Severe depression, risk of suicide/self-neglect or other serious risk	Antidepressant, combined treatments, Electroconvulsive therapy

etine), beginning with a low dose and gradually titrating up to the maximum, depending upon response. It is recommended that sufficient time is left between increases to allow the drug to begin working because it is considered that the therapeutic effect usually takes about two to three weeks to manifest.

If, after a few weeks at the maximum dose, the patient continues to complain of symptoms of depression and other CMDs, the drug should be slowly reduced over a period of weeks. At each review, it is prudent to ask whether the patient is actually taking the drug and make a rapid assessment of the mental state to ascertain if things are improving anyway.

Continued use of illicit drugs (cocaine, ecstasy, crack etc.) and alcohol are unlikely to help the patient's mental state and regular review of their use is important.

An alternative medication from another class should then be introduced and again the dose slowly titrated up to the maximum, allowing plenty of time between increments for the therapeutic action to commence. Use of the tricyclics (e.g. amitryptyline, imipramine) or venlafaxine, should, according to NICE, be second line in more severe cases. Currently, psychiatrists are combining venlafaxine and mirtazepine after first and second line antidepressants have failed. Such a combination should be under the supervision of a psychiatrist.

Mood stabilisers, combinations and other agents

The prescription of lithium and anticonvulsants, used either alone or in combination with other psychotropic agents, should be embarked upon only with advice and support from psychiatrists. Also, combining antidepressants and antipsychotic drugs should not be attempted without direction from doctors in secondary care. As noted above, the NICE guidelines do not recommend the use of hypnotics or anxiolytics in the treatment of CMDs because of the problem of dependence. If insomnia is a particularly dominant complaint in the patient's presentation, then a sedative antidepressant should be chosen e.g. mirtazepine or amitryptyline.

Psychological treatments

Introduction

GPs regularly use psychotherapeutic skills whether or not they intentionally employ them. They use them every day of their professional lives to deal with almost all of their patients. The phrase: 'The doctor as drug' remains as important to primary care today as it did when first coined by Balint more than 40 years ago (1964). All doctors have probably experienced prescribing a medication and having the patient come back a day or two later saying: 'I didn't take the tablets because I felt much better as soon as I'd talked to you'.

Counselling

Counselling is a broad term used in mental health services to mean therapeutic counselling. It is an umbrella expression which covers psychotherapy services. It is generally accepted to mean a form of talking therapy which is short and oriented towards helping patients use their own resources to resolve problems of a less severe nature.

Time spent sourcing names and addresses of all counselling services available locally can save valuable clinic minutes during the course of a busy surgery.

The following organisations are given by way of example; they are both national organisations and one has local branches throughout the country. Other counselling services may be available for specific problems commonly encountered in local areas and it is worth making contact with them.

MIND (http://www.mind.org.uk/)

The organisation provides many different services including crisis helplines, drop-in centres, counselling, befriending, advocacy, employment and training schemes.

SANE (http://www.sane.org.uk/)

SANE provides supportive counselling over the phone or via its new email service SANEmail.

For more complicated cases, crisis intervention services and psychological treatments in its various forms are preferred options.

Crisis Intervention Services

The roots of crisis intervention come from the pioneering work of two community psychiatrists – Erich Lindemann and Gerald Caplan in the mid-1940s, 1950s and 1960s.

Caplan was the first clinician to describe and document the four stages of a crisis reaction:

1. The initial rise of tension from the emotionally hazardous, crisis-precipitating event
2. Increasing disruption of daily living because the individual is stuck and cannot resolve the crisis quickly
3. Tension rapidly increases as the individual fails to resolve the crisis through emergency problem-solving methods
4. The person goes into a depression or mental collapse, or may partially resolve the crisis by using new coping methods

Psychological treatments

The most common schools of psychotherapy are cognitive behavioural therapy (CBT), psychoanalytic (also called psychodynamic) psychotherapy and systemic therapy. See Chapter 18 for more information.

As a simple rule of thumb, CBT has been shown to be better than placebo in the treatment of moderate disease (depression and the mixture of anxiety and depression).

For disease at the milder end of the spectrum, CBT has no real benefit over watching and waiting. Moderate to severe disease may respond to CBT, where it has been shown to be better than placebo or medication. For the more severe case, antidepressant medication is the treatment of choice.

Other treatments

Cognitive behavioural therapy programmes delivered online or on-screen (known as computerised CBT or cCBT) have been used to treat mild and moderate depressive illness with some degree of success.

Stress management courses have been shown to be effective in the management of generalised anxiety disorder and mild depressive disorders with an anxiety component.

Exercise has also been shown to be effective to counteract mild depressive illness, or low mood, and many patients will put their need to regularly attend the gym to keep them 'well' as evidence of pathology.

St John's Wort has also been used to treat depressive disorders for many years. The evidence for its effect is not convincing.

Prognosis and outcome

Two out of five patients presenting with common mental illness in general practice (even when considered ill enough to merit psychiatric input) improve rapidly within a few weeks. Thirty per cent pursue a slower course to recovery, which leaves a remaining 30% who have a poor prognosis with frequent relapses – see Figure 2.4.

A recent study reported similar results. Approximately 60% of depressed patients had a good outcome, 30% had a fluctuating outcome and 10% had a poor outcome, remaining depressed over a six month follow-up period. In essence, 20–30% of depressed patients have a poor outcome, either suffering long-term sickness or having a relapsing fluctuating state.

Factors predicting a good outcome have been found to include an early response to treatments and a low level of personality disorder symptoms. Figures for the incidence of suicide vary from about 15% down to 2.2%.

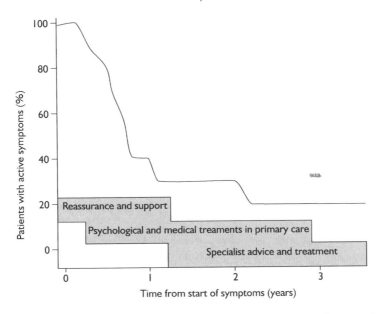

Figure 2.4 Resolution of new onset neurotic disorders (from Craig and Board-man, 1997).

Personality disorder, drugs, alcohol, physical symptoms and comorbidity (dual diagnosis)

Personality disorder

An understanding of a patient's personality or make-up is extremely helpful in the assessment and treatment of all primary care patients. It will have a bearing on both their physical and mental health. With regard to depression and its associated disorders it has an effect on prognosis.

The idea of a personality disorder is again, like unhappiness, an artificial distinction between normal and abnormal. Psychiatrists have defined it as:

A severe disturbance in the characterological constitution and behavioural tendencies of the individual, usually involving several areas of the personality, and nearly always associated with considerable personal and social disruption

Personality disorder tends to appear in late childhood or adolescence and continues to be manifest into adulthood. It is therefore unlikely that the diagnosis of personality disorder will be appropriate before the age of 16 or 17 years.

Drugs and alcohol

The importance of assessing the use of drugs and alcohol in patients suffering from depression and its associated disorders cannot be overemphasised. Continued use (or abuse) of a substance may lead to a degree of dependence. In this situation, it may be that the dependency is the problem and the psychiatric or psychological problem is simply secondary to it. Psychologically based treatments, like psycho-analytical psychotherapy, need the patient to be sober and free from withdrawal symptoms in order for them to have an effect on the patient's mental state.

Physical symptoms and disease

Sufferers of depression may complain of somatic symptoms as part of their presentation. In fact, as already noted, about two-thirds of depressed patients mainly complain of physical problems. In some cases, psychiatrists may diagnose a somatoform disorder (somatisation disorder or hypochondriasis) or rarely some form of dissociative disorder (also known as conversion or hysterical reactions). Certainly, research has shown that more than half of patients with an anxiety or depressive disorder fulfilled the criteria for a comorbid somatoform disorder.

Patients with these conditions usually resist attempts to discuss the possibility of psychological causation even when the onset and continuation of the symptoms bear a close relationship with unpleasant life events, difficulties or conflicts.

The future

The assessment and treatment of depression and its associated disorders is difficult. GPs have been unfairly criticised for many failings with regard to diagnosis and treatment of the condition over the past twenty years. Screening tools, guidelines and protocols have been used in an effort to improve the situation. However, mainly due to the nature of the illnesses themselves the effects of such measures have been limited. Indeed, a landmark study of repeated measures of health, disability and satisfaction at follow-up failed to find any significant differences between practices using guidelines and practices giving usual care. And further, contrary to expectation, the guideline practices achieved higher average disability scores, indicating worse outcome; they did achieve greater satisfaction with care received, but this was associated with worse quality of life (Croudace *et al.*, 2003).

The publication of guidelines on the treatment of depression by NICE have also been criticised for failing to recommend an approach based on a chronic disease management model.

As has been mentioned above, the symptoms of patients suffering from CMDs cannot be easily or clearly separated from normal thoughts, behaviours and emotions; and therein is a problem for the GP being asked to treat them. Screening tools, guidelines and educational programmes for the beleaguered practitioner have been found wanting even though they have been universally adopted as the *modus operandi* of assessing and managing CMDs. Such a bewildering state of affairs becomes even more confusing when the latest NICE guidelines continue to recommend treatments (both pharmacological and psychological) which are probably ineffective (Kirsch *et al.*, 2008; Lynch *et al.*, 2009).

Further, by looking again at the outcome data for CMDs, it can be appreciated that more than 40% of them will resolve in a couple of months; a figure which reaches approximately 70% by 12 months. More likely than not, some psychiatrists (and no doubt some GPs) would have diagnosed many of the patients who improved in the short term as suffering from adjustment disorders; in essence they would have concluded that the patients had developed a variety of symptoms (including unhappiness and anxiety) as a result of a stressful event. The question which follows then is: 'Can an adjustment disorder be distinguished from depression and the other CMDs?'. The matter has been the subject of much debate and research and remains unresolved, although evidence points towards the two conditions being indistinguishable (Casey *et al.*, 2006).

Turning now to the remaining 30% who continue to experience symptoms by the end of the 12 months, it should be appreciated that research has found that their long-term outlook is poor (Merikangas *et al.*, 2003). The type or make-up of the patient's personality undoubtedly plays a major role in accounting for such a depressing prognosis. Hence, any treatment for this group must involve long-term intensive psychological therapy or combinations of antidepressants and mood stabilisers or both. Successful treatment outcomes of such patients are rare.

In summary, deciding who to treat and which treatment or treatments to use in attenders complaining of symptoms of CMDs at general practice surgeries is complicated. The task is made even more problematic given the time constraints under which GPs are working.

Pragmatically, the group causing primary care physicians most concern is that for whom two or three antidepressants have been prescribed without success. Such a situation usually arises after several months and, as noted above, once the symptoms have been present for 12 months or more the prognosis becomes poorer and poorer. Needless to say, the GP should still continue to try different treatments. Indeed, miraculous improvements have been achieved in some patients using mixtures of different antidepressants augmented with various mood stabilisers or with long-term psychological treatments or combinations of both modalities. Such treatments need input from secondary care services.

Finally, GPs (and all doctors for that matter) need to be aware of the limitations of modern medicine. Some diseases (including those with poorly defined symptoms) are not treatable. In such cases the physician experiences understandable frustration and annoyance – here more than ever, care, consideration and empathy need to be shown to the patient.

Improving access to psychological therapies

An ambitious plan to increase the availability of psychological therapy for patients suffering from depression and other CMDs was launched by the UK Government in 2007. The project, led by the eminent economist Richard Layard, involves training approximately 10,000 therapists over a seven year period. The policy, based on NICE guidelines, aims to reduce waiting times for CBT and provide treatment to all patients requesting it. The plan has not been universally accepted as a panacea to the problem of treating increasing numbers of patients suffering from depression and other CMDs. Critics fear that the growing medicalisation of societal distress will reach epidemic proportions.

Conclusion

Up-to-date evidence points towards the use of a chronic care model for the management of depression. Such a model would be multifaceted and flexible so as to provide a level of support dependent upon results. It necessitates the close monitoring of patients over the whole course of the illness, allowing treatments to be stepped up or stepped down. Excessive or inappropriate treatments for patients should thereby be avoided and the provision of more complex intensive interventions should only be provided for those requiring them. Clearly such a plan is not without financial implications.

In an ideal world no one would become depressed or anxious. The World Health Organization has produced much literature on the promotion of mental health and the prevention of illness. It has recently published a series of articles on the matter under the mantra: 'There is no health without mental health'. For further details, the interested reader is advised to follow the link below to the WHO website:

http://www.who.int/topics/mental_health/en/

Key points

- Depression and mixed anxiety and depression are the two most common psychiatric conditions seen in primary care.
- Ninety per cent of all psychological and psychiatric illnesses are dealt with by general practitioners.
- Under-diagnosis and under-treatment of psychological and psychiatric illness often occur in primary care.
- The effectiveness of current treatments, including antidepressants and cognitive behavioural therapy, has been questioned in recent meta-analyses.
- Depression and other common mental disorders are best managed and treated under the chronic care model using a case-managed, multidisciplinary team approach.

Further reading and bibliography

Balint, M. (1964) *The Doctor, His Patient and the Illness.* Pitman Medical, London.

Casey. P., Maracy, M., Kelly, B. D., Lehtinen, V., Ayuso-Mateos, J. L., Dalgard, O. S. and Dowrick, C. (2006) Can adjustment disorder and depressive episode be distinguished? Results from ODIN. *Journal of Affective Disorders*, **92**, 291–7.

Craig, T. K. and Boardman, A. P. (1997) ABC of mental health. Common mental health problems in primary care. *British Medical Journal*, **314**, 1609–12.

Croudace, T., Evans, J., Harrison, G., Sharp, D. J., Wilkinson, E., McCann, G., Spence, M., Crilly, C. and Brindle, L. (2003) Impact of the ICD-10 Primary Health Care (PHC) diagnostic and management guidelines for mental disorders on detection and outcome in primary care. Cluster randomised controlled trial. *British Journal of Psychiatry*, **182**, 20–30.

Kessler, D., Lloyd, K., Lewis, G. and Gray, D. P. (1999) Cross-sectional study of symptom attribution and recognition of depression and anxiety in primary care. *British Medical Journal*, **318**, 436–9.

Kirsch, I., Deacon, B. J., Huedo-Medina, T. B., Scoboria, A., Moore, T. J. and Johnson, B. T. (2008) Initial severity and antidepressant benefits: a meta-analysis of data submitted to the Food and Drug Administration. *PLoS Medicine*, **5**, e45.

Lynch, D., Laws, K. R., and McKenna, P. J. (2009) Cognitive behavioural therapy for major psychiatric disorder: does it really work? A meta-analytical review of well-controlled trials. *Psychological Medicine*, **40**, 9–24.

Merikangas, K. R., Zhang, H., Avenevoli, S., Acharyya, S., Neuenschwander, M. and Angst, J. (2003) Longitudinal trajectories of depression and anxiety in a prospective community study: the Zurich Cohort Study. *Archives of General Psychiatry*, **60**, 993–1000.

NICE (2004) *Anxiety: Management of Anxiety (Panic Disorder, with or Without Agoraphobia, and General Anxiety Disorder) in Adults in Primary, Secondary and Community Care*. Clinical guidelines CG22. National Institute for Health and Clinical Excellence, London. http://guidance.nice.org.uk/CG22.

NICE (2009) *The Treatment and Management of Depression in Adults (Update)*. Clinical guidelines CG90. National Institute for Health and Clinical Excellence, London. http://guidance.nice.org.uk/CG90.

CHAPTER 3

Severe mental illness

Kazuya Iwata

Case history 1

A 32-year-old female presents to her GP requesting a brain scan. According to her, she has been implanted with an electronic device by God and has been receiving messages. She is now requesting a scan as she finds these messages to be loud and wants the volume adjusted.

Her friend reports that she has been acting strangely for the last four months and has recently lost her job. Her medical history is unremarkable and there is no history of any illicit substance use.

Case history 2

A 20-year-old male is brought to his GP by his mother, who is becoming increasingly concerned about her son's bizarre behaviour and significant weight loss over the last six months. The patient claims that the food and tap water in his house are poisoned, and has been surviving on minimal takeaway food bought by his parents, which he reluctantly eats after hours of persuasion. He is housebound due to lack of energy and looks pale and wasted.

His mother reports that he used to smoke cannabis when he was 15 years old but has not used any illicit substances since then.

Case history 3

A 28-year-old female is referred to her GP by her workplace as she has been loud and disruptive at work for over a week. The patient does not feel that there is any problem, as she feels that she is just being friendly to her customers and has been inventing innovative ways of working. She has not slept for four days as she has been trying to draft a report on how to solve global warming. On mental state examination, she is overactive and unable to sit still. She is irritable when questioned in detail, and answers in a loud voice.

Her past history is significant of a depressive illness, which was treated successfully by her GP with an antidepressant. She is currently not on any medication.

Introduction

Severe mental illness (SMI) refers to a group of illnesses characterised by the presence of psychosis. *Psychosis* is a general term used to define symptoms which are qualitatively different from normal experiences, most commonly represented by delusions (fixed beliefs not in line with the person's background) and hallucinations (abnormal perceptions occurring in the absence of an actual stimuli, seen in all modalities). Psychosis is a key feature of schizophrenia (and associated illnesses such as schizoaffective disorder and delusional disorders) and severe affective disorders (psychotic depression and bipolar affective disorder), although psychotic symptoms can manifest in some personality disorders, organic illnesses and substance misuse. Severe mental illness usually refers to schizophrenia-type disorders and bipolar affective disorder.

Schizophrenia

Schizophrenia is a psychotic illness in which the patient's sense of reality is lost, with symptoms leading to deterioration in their social functioning. These symptoms include not only delusions and hallucinations, but also inappropriate affect, thought disorder (manifesting as disorganised speech), cognitive impairment and negativism. It affects roughly 1% of the population and has an equal sex distribution, although the onset is earlier in males (early twenties, as opposed to late twenties in female). Schizophrenia can manifest in different subtypes (such as paranoid and hebephrenic), and its key symptoms are summarised in Table 3.1.

Table 3.1 Key symptoms of severe mental illness.

Schizophrenia	Bipolar affective disorder
Paranoid schizophrenia ■ Persistent delusions that are not culturally appropriate or are implausible ■ Hallucinations, usually auditory (third person commentary) or in other modalities	*Mania* ■ Increased energy, leading to overactivity and reduced sleep ■ Increased distractibility and irritability ■ Increased pressure of speech due to racing thoughts ■ Increased self-esteem and grandiosity ■ Increase in risk-taking behaviours, such as overspending and recklessness
Hebephrenic schizophrenia ■ Thought disorder, manifesting as disorganised speech ■ Flat or inappropriate affect	*Hypomania* ■ Manic symptoms, but milder ■ Difficulty focusing on one task ■ Overfamiliarity ■ Increased sex drive ■ Sociability and talkativeness
Catatonic schizophrenia ■ Immobile, or agitated and repetitive movements	
Simple schizophrenia ■ Negative symptoms such as apathy and reduced motivation	

Bipolar affective disorder

Bipolar affective disorder is an affective disorder defined by the presence of abnormally elevated or depressed mood. It is thought to affect between 0.3 and 1.5% of the population, affecting both sexes equally, with the first onset usually starting in early adulthood (peaking at 15–19 years and 20–24 years old). Its core feature is mania, which refers to a state of elevated mood lasting for more than one week, with symptoms severe enough to cause substantial social disruption. These symptoms can usually reach psychotic levels, whereby the person may start forming grandiose delusions, such as the belief that they possess special powers. On the other hand, hypomania refers to a cluster of symptoms which are milder and less socially disruptive than mania. Table 3.1 summarises the key symptoms seen in mania and hypomania. At least two episodes of mood disturbance, one of which must be of mania or hypomania, are required for a diagnosis of bipolar affective disorder.

For both schizophrenia and bipolar affective disorder, a family history does increase one's susceptibility, although the effects of genetic loading are thought to be greater in bipolar affective disorder. However, the aetiology of these illnesses is multifactorial and it is often very difficult to elucidate one single causative agent.

History

A patient with severe mental illness presenting to the GP may not necessarily present with complaints about their delusions or hallucinations. Rather, they are usually brought in by their family, carers or friends, who become increasingly concerned about the individual's change in behaviour and presentation.

As with any other patient, a history of the chief complaint should be obtained from the patient, focusing on what the actual nature of the complaint is and how this is affecting them. Any potential key events which may have triggered the complaint should be obtained. This needs to be done sensitively, as excessive confrontation of the patient's delusions or psychotic experiences can affect the therapeutic relationship and may make further management difficult.

Collateral history is of great value in assessing patients with a severe mental illness, especially as the nature of the psychotic symptoms usually prevents patients from having an insight into their illness. As a result, history from friends and carers allows accurate depiction of the sequence of events, leading to the current presentation and how the patient has been coping so far.

Other aspects of the history that would be useful in ascertaining the problem include the following:

- Previous contacts with psychiatric services
- Medication history, especially psychiatric medications and responses achieved
- Use of illicit substances – stimulants (e.g. amphetamines, cocaine), hallucinogens (e.g. LSD, ketamine) and cannabis can cause psychosis or changes in mood. Drug-induced psychosis should be excluded before making a diagnosis of schizophrenia or bipolar affective disorder. However, drug use frequently occurs concurrently, and can complicate the presentation, delay recovery (persistent symptoms) and increase the risk of relapse

Mental state examination

The mental state examination focuses on the snapshot picture of the patient's mental state at the time of presentation, and allows one to keep track of the change in patient's symptoms. This is important in assessing severe mental illness as it allows one to examine the severity of the symptoms. The following points need to be identified when assessing the mental state.

Appearance and behaviour

Is the patient's attire appropriate? Are there signs of neglect? Is the patient showing signs of severe agitation or retardation? Any abnormal behaviour, such as repetitive motions? Does the patient appear guarded and suspicious, or are they overly familiar?

Speech

Disorder of the patient's thought form is reflected in their speech, and this is seen in both schizophrenia and bipolar affective disorder. Loosening of association occurs when the patient's ideas or sentences do not have any connection and their response as a whole does not make sense. When the sentence is composed of random words stuck together without any association, this is called word salad. This may also be associated with neologism, where the patient creates a new word.

Commonly in mania flight of ideas is seen, whereby the patient skips topics midway through the conversation as ideas are racing in their heads. Their speech may also be pressured and difficult to interrupt. On the other hand, in a severely depressed state, the patient may present with lack of spontaneity and may not speak much (poverty of thought).

Mood and affect

Changes in mood are a core feature of affective disorders, and in bipolar affective disorder patients present in an excited and expansive mood when in a manic phase. This can be accompanied by irritability, or even a volatile switch of their emotions (labile affect). The opposite is true when the patient is in a severely depressed state, in that they retain a mask-like facial expression without much change to their emotions (blunted affect).

Thought

In severe mental illness, the thought content may be held at delusional intensity, whereby the beliefs are unshakeable and represent the 'truth' to the patient. The delusions are usually paranoid, in that the beliefs have some connection to them. The commonest paranoid delusion is that of persecution, where the patient feels that they are being followed, conspired against or cheated by an external agency or person. Other types of delusion include grandiose (for example having special powers – this is commonly seen in mania), erotomania (someone, usually a celebrity or someone of high social class, is in love with them), religious, and of control (that someone or something is controlling their body and behaviour).

Abnormal experiences

Hallucinations are seen in both schizophrenia and bipolar affective disorder, and the commonest modality is auditory. These need to be occurring outside the head (as if someone is talking to them) in order to be considered a frank hallucinatory experience. The content of these hallucinations can vary, ranging from derogatory, commanding and religious to non-speech like sounds (such as gun shots). Hallucinations can also occur in other modalities, such as visual (e.g. neighbour spying on them on the fifth floor balcony), olfactory (e.g. skin rotting) and tactile (e.g. feeling like someone is touching them).

Cognition and insight

The presence of psychosis usually prevents the patient from having a full insight into their illness, and those who are presenting with these symptoms for the first time will usually not be able to link their symptoms with having a mental illness.

Risk

The presence of delusions and hallucinations can be distressing to the patient and/or others, and a thorough assessment of their risk needs to be undertaken. A full history, together with an assessment of their mental state, should inform the level of risk they pose to themselves and others, and indicate the urgency of referral to secondary services.

Physical examination and investigation

A physical examination, including a neurological examination, is necessary to rule out a neurological lesion. Diagnosis of a severe mental illness is dependent on the patient's history and mental state examination, and therefore there are no confirmatory investigations available. However, it is important to rule out any organic causes and thus a baseline blood test (to include full blood count, renal function, liver function, calcium and glucose) is required.

Management

The management of patients presenting with a suspected case of severe mental illness usually requires referral to secondary services, and early intervention is advised to prevent a deterioration in their mental state. The type of secondary services required depends largely on the severity of the symptoms and the risks the patients pose to themselves and others.

In secondary services, the patient's care plan will comprise of medication, psychological therapies and/or social interventions. It will be important for the GP to obtain copies of the care plan and institute them accordingly. A large proportion of those with severe mental illness will be placed on a Care Programme Approach (CPA) and may be allocated a community case worker. It is essential to engage the patient, where possible, in a therapeutic alliance. This involves providing information on the nature of their illness, its course and prognosis, the benefits and side-effects of treatment (pharmacological and non-pharmacological), factors associated with relapse (non-compliance with medication and impact of continuing drug use) and discussion of early indicators of relapse, and what they should do in the event of a crisis. The views of the patient and their carers should be taken into account when recommending treatment options, and patients should be encouraged to take responsibility for their treatment.

Schizophrenia

All patients presenting with psychotic symptoms suggestive of schizophrenia-type illness should be referred to secondary services for a comprehensive assessment and formulation of a care plan. The type of secondary service that the patient should be referred to will depend on the urgency of the situation (the level of risk to the patient or others), and other factors such as age and local availability (see Chapter 13).

If there are concerns about the patient's level of risk or severity of symptoms, an urgent inpatient admission may need to be arranged. If he or she is willing to be admitted informally, then a referral to the Crisis Resolution or Home Treatment Team should be made (either directly or via the duty psychiatrist). They will assess the patient for suitability for home treatment or inpatient admission. If the patient is refusing an informal admission, a Mental Health Act assessment may need to be arranged by the GP (see Chapter 16). Features in the history or presentation that suggest an urgent referral include:

- Risk of harm to self (self-harm, suicide or threats from others); e.g. voices instructing them to kill themselves
- Risk of harm to others (particularly if specific threats are being made towards an individual and there is access to weapons); e.g. due to persecutory delusions or delusions of control
- Risk of self-neglect – e.g. not eating or drinking due to beliefs about food contamination or being poisoned, or severe withdrawal
- Catatonic symptoms (rare) – mutism, stupor or motor excitement

For non-urgent situations, a referral should be made to the local Community Mental Health Team (CMHT). If this is the patient's first presentation and he or she is under the age of 35, a referral to the Early Intervention Service may be appropriate (see Chapter 13).

In treating patients with schizophrenia, the medication regime will usually be initiated by the psychiatrist in secondary services. The regime will usually consist of an antipsychotic medication, usually an oral atypical antipsychotic. However, in patients where compliance may be problem, this may be converted to a depot injection medication in the long term.

On some occasions, it may be necessary for the GP to initiate antipsychotic treatment while waiting for the patient to be seen by secondary services. In these cases, this should be undertaken by GPs with experience in treating schizophrenia and following discussion with the community Consultant Psychiatrist. The choice of antipsychotic will need to be made after having discussed the risks and benefits with the patient.

Bipolar affective disorder

For patients with bipolar affective disorder, the decision to refer to secondary services will depend largely on their presentation. Patients presenting with mania or severe depression who are a risk to themselves (self-harm, suicide, risk of sexual or financial exploitation, self-neglect) or risk to others, are likely to require an inpatient admission and should be referred urgently to the Crisis Resolution Team or the local CMHT. Other patients who are presenting with prolonged overactive, disinhibited behaviours (suggestive of hypomania) with repeated periods of depressive episodes should be referred to the CMHT for assessment and formulation of a care plan.

If a new patient with existing bipolar affective disorder registers with the practice, a referral to secondary services should be considered.

The medical treatment of bipolar affective disorder comprises of atypical antipsychotics (such as olanzapine) and/or mood stabilisers, such as sodium valproate and lithium. Antidepressants are also used in cases where the predominant illness is depressive, but caution needs to be exercised as this may swing the patient into a manic state. Therefore the treatment of depressive symptoms in bipolar affective disorder is usually through the optimisation of mood stabilisers. A time-limited trial of benzodiazepines for the short term may be considered where behavioural disturbance such as agitation continues to present as a problem.

Medication

Antipsychotics

Antipsychotics are used in treating both schizophrenia and mania, but to a greater extent in schizophrenia. The current guidelines advocate the use of atypical antipsychotics as the first line treatment of schizophrenia. Commonly used atypicals include quetiapine, olanzapine and risperidone.

Both the typical and atypical antipsychotics do have the propensity to cause side-effects, most notably extra-pyramidal side-effects (EPSEs). These include akathisia (inner restlessness), dystonia (muscle spasms), parkinsonism and tardive dyskinesia (involuntary irregular muscle movements, usually of the face – they are irreversible once they develop). EPSEs can be treated with anticholinergic medication such as procyclidine and orphenadrine.

Metabolic side-effects are also seen more commonly with atypicals, and they are associated with an increased risk of hyperglycaemia, hypertension, central obesity and hyperlipidaemia. See Chapter 17 for further information.

Mood stabilisers

Mood stabilisers are used in treating bipolar affective disorder. In the treatment of hypomania or mania, lithium or valproate are used, although valproate needs to be avoided in women of childbearing age due to its teratogenic effects. See Chapter 17 for further information.

Monitoring of mental and physical health

It is important to note that patients with a severe mental illness tend to engage less with their GPs and thus a proactive approach in monitoring their physical and mental health needs to be taken. In the community, patients should be reviewed routinely by GPs for their mental state, and they should be referred to secondary care services urgently if acute exacerbation of their psychiatric symptoms is noted or response to treatment is poor.

Patients with a severe mental illness do suffer from higher mortality and morbidity compared to the general population, and thus regular screening of their physical health is required. Their poor physical health can be attributed to various factors, including a sedentary lifestyle, but the side-effects of the psychotropic medication also do need to be borne in mind.

A yearly blood test is required for patients with severe mental illness, and this should cover the following:

- *If on antipsychotics*: Full blood count, renal function, liver function, glucose, lipid profile
- *If on mood stabilisers, including lithium*: As for antipsychotics, but also to include thyroid function tests and lithium levels. If the patient's lithium level exceeds 1.2 mmol/L, the patient will need to be referred to secondary services at once to prevent lithium toxicity. At levels over 1.5 mmol/L, the patient may start experiencing symptoms of toxicity and will require urgent medical attention.

Patients should also have their blood pressure and weight measured at the same time.

Some patients with severe schizophrenia will be treated with clozapine, which requires registration with the Clozaril Patient Monitoring Service (CPMS). This medication can only be commenced in secondary services and these patients will require blood testing (for white blood cell count), which will usually be coordinated by the secondary services. Special care needs to be taken if these patients present with symptoms such as sore a throat, as the most worrying side-effect of clozapine is agranulocytosis and thus if this is suspected, they will need to stop clopazine and be referred to secondary services at once.

Other treatment options

Psychosocial interventions are also useful in the treatment of severe mental illness, in particular to help patients understand and cope with their illnesses. Cognitive behavioural therapy (CBT) is a time-limited intervention that focuses on treating current symptoms, and it can be used to educate patients about their illness (such as recognising relapse indicators), teaching coping skills with psychosocial stressors, facilitating compliance with their treatment, and restoring self-confidence. These can ultimately be structured as part of relapse prevention work.

Family therapy addresses the family as a whole and has been found to be beneficial, especially in educating the family about the illness and helping them deal with the consequences. In this way, potential stress within the family can be kept to a minimum, thereby preventing the patient from being exposed to any emotional outbursts within the family (expressed emotion).

Other treatment options include support groups, which are usually run by the voluntary sector and are helpful in patients structuring their days, meeting fellow patients, and receiving support in getting vocational training. Occupational therapy is also used routinely to help assess patients' activities of daily living skills so that they may be able to regain the living skills they may have lost through their illness.

Key points

- A comprehensive history and mental state examination, including obtaining collateral information, is crucial in order to understand the patient's presentation given the communication difficulties associated with severe mental illness.
- All patients presenting with schizophrenia-type illness need to be referred to secondary services urgently, so that early treatment and a care plan can be instituted.
- Urgent referral is required for patients with mania or severe depressive episode who are at risk to themselves or others. Other patients with bipolar affective disorder should be referred to secondary services to formulate a comprehensive care plan.
- A yearly review of physical health for patients with severe mental illness needs to be carried out in primary care. This should include blood tests and measurements of weight and blood pressure.
- Even when under the care of secondary services, patients will need to be reviewed routinely by their GPs in the community. If there are changes in symptoms or an acute exacerbation of their presentation occurs, they will need to be referred urgently to secondary services.

Further reading and bibliography

Gelder, M., Mayou, R. and Cowen, P. (2001) *Shorter Oxford Textbook of Psychiatry*. Oxford University Press, New York.

NICE (2006) *The Management of Bipolar Disorder in Adults, Children and Adolescents, in Primary and Secondary Care*. Clinical guidelines CG38. National Institute for Health and Clinical Excellence, London. http://guidance.nice.org.uk/CG38.

NICE (2009) *Core Interventions in the Treatment and Management of Schizophrenia in Adults in Primary and Secondary Care (Update)*. Clinical guidelines CG82. National Institute for Health and Clinical Excellence, London. http://guidance. nice.org.uk/CG82.

Semple, D., Smyth, R., Burns, J., Darjee, R. and McIntosh, A. (2005), *Oxford Handbook of Psychiatry*. Oxford University Press, New York.

CHAPTER 4

Alcohol and substance misuse

Vanessa Crawford and Lucy Carter

Case history

A 35-year-old man attends your surgery requesting a methadone prescription. He is using crack cocaine and heroin daily and has done for months; he is now injecting into the groin. You notice the smell of alcohol when he has left the room. He says that he wants to get 'clean' so that he can see his children again. He is defensive when asked about his criminal history. He does not want to go to the local specialist NHS drug service, as he went there 10 years ago and didn't like the 'regime'. He mentions in passing that his girlfriend is pregnant.

Introduction

According to the Royal College of General Practitioners the prevalence of drug problems is 42 per 1000 cases per week; this is equal to the number of depressive episodes per week seen in general practice. Alcohol problems are seen in 81 per 1000 cases per week. Given these figures, are we doing enough to screen for drug and alcohol problems? A complex, polydrug user in the 21st century is better nourished, has easier access to drugs and is more likely to become pregnant than a drug user 20 years ago. The profile of those who use substances has changed markedly over the last two decades; the prevalence and range of drugs used has increased significantly. The combination of drugs used by individuals has also become more complex, requiring a greater knowledge of the individual drugs and their interactions.

Assessment

History taking

It is important to establish what the patient is looking for from the consultation, but be upfront with the patient that they will not necessarily get a prescription that day. Praise him or her for taking the first step to change and use a non-judgemental style of questioning: 'this may not apply to you but I want to ask you some questions about drugs and alcohol that can cause health problems'.

Current patterns of drug usage

Enquire about current drug and alcohol use over the last four weeks. It is useful to name specific drugs, as the patient may not disclose all their drug use if not asked. Do not forget to ask about cigarettes and alcohol.

Ask how much they use each drug (in weight or money), how often and by which route they administer it (oral, intranasal, subcutaneous, intramuscular, intravenous, rectal).

Enquire about what the benefits and disadvantages of drug use are and the effects if they are not able to use the drug (withdrawal symptoms). Ask how long they can go without and when the last period of abstinence was and how they achieved it. Is there any history of delirium tremens, seizures, substance related hospitalisation, and intentional or unintentional overdose?

Ask about current risks – the nature of drug use, do they live with or have contact with children (does there appear to be a risk to the children from emotional and/or physical abuse or neglect?), and are there any protective influences. Be clear from the outset about your duty of care to the patient and to third parties if the patient is threatening to harm them. If he or she has a partner, are they also using drugs? Enquire whether social services are already involved and if this is why he or she wants to 'become clean' now?

Medical history

Ask general and specific questions about substance-related physical illnesses such as DVT, skin abscesses, cellulitis, wheezing (crack and heroin use), endocarditis, viral hepatitis and HIV status. Bear in mind illnesses such as TB, which has become more prevalent in recent times and is particularly associated with crack cocaine use within clusters of individuals.

Psychiatric history

- Are they depressed or anxious?
- Any abnormal thoughts/psychosis?
- Any suicidal thoughts? Any active plans to end their life?
- Any admissions under a psychiatrist?
- Currently on any antidepressant or antipsychotic medication?
- Have they ever been on medication for mental illness?

Criminal history in brief

Have they ever been in trouble with the police or had to do sex work to fund their habit?

Social support

What are their current social circumstances and what support do they need?
Are they in stable housing or receiving social security benefits? How do they spend their days – are there any interests, hobbies, employment or qualifications they may want to pursue? Are there local organisations that could help them with this?

Mental state examination

What is their current presentation? Are they distressed, depressed or suicidal? Is their thinking clear and coherent? Are they experiencing any psychotic phenomena? Do they have any thoughts of harming others? Is there a sense of cognitive impairment even if not fully tested?

Physical examination

This must be carried out before the patient leaves. Look at their general physical state, including dentition (if possible). Examine for the presence of any ulcers or cellulitis on their legs or at injection sites. Check their temperature. Look for signs of injecting drug use; this may be hidden to avoid detection by others (e.g. groin or leg injecting so that the family does not notice). Look at the quality of the injecting sites to see how good the technique is.

Examine for signs of liver disease; there seems to be a much greater tendency for individuals to deny excessive alcohol use than to deny their drug use. It may therefore be necessary to utilise the findings of blood tests (gamma glutamyl transferase, liver function tests, mean corpuscular volume) and findings on physical examination to feed back to the patient that they may be drinking to an extent where it is affecting their health. Look for stigmata of endocarditis – e.g. fever, splinter haemorrhages, murmurs or signs of deep venous thrombosis (calf swelling, pain).

Have a listen to their chest and do a peak flow, which may be reduced if they are smoking crack cocaine or heroin regularly. Are they wheezing? Do they have signs of pneumonia or TB?

Investigations

Alcohol screening tools

The Alcohol Use Disorders Identification Test (AUDIT) can be used to identify patients with hazardous and harmful patterns of alcohol consumption. The AUDIT was developed by the World Health Organization (WHO) as a simple method of screening for excessive drinking and to assist in a brief assessment and can help in identifying excessive drinking as the cause of the presenting illness. It also provides a framework for intervention to help hazardous and harmful drinkers reduce or cease alcohol consumption and thereby avoid the harmful consequences of their drinking. It can be used as an interview or self-report tool.

It is very important to warn patients about the significant risks associated with their drinking and combined substance use. There is often a request for repeated alcohol detoxification; there is evidence that this can be harmful in terms of precipitating seizures and exacerbating cognitive impairment. Liver failure may also be noted on detoxification; it is unclear whether this is the stress of detoxification or the unmasking of something present already.

Drug screening

Urine should be obtained for drug screening (ask the laboratory for full drugs of misuse screen); be aware that drug tests vary in their cut-off levels for a positive test, so there is no absolute formula for predicting when a drug was last used. 6-monoacetylmorphine is one of the most useful tests in this respect as it demonstrates heroin use within 8 hours of the test sample being taken.

Urine drug screens sent to the laboratory may take up to a week to return to the GP. However, some GP practices may have on-the-spot urine drug testing, or the local Community Drug Team may do on the spot drug screening.

Mouth swabs can be used to test for drug use when urine cannot be produced or there is concern as to the origin of the urine (patients can dilute their urine or bring someone else's sample). If there is doubt about the authenticity of the sample, walk the patient to the bathroom and give them a new pot clearly labelled by you.

Hair tests can be arranged directly by social services if they need to look at longitudinal drug use for child protection purposes.

However, one positive test does not establish dependence; a good history, examination and the option of a second test after three days make the diagnosis more robust.

Blood tests

Blood tests should include a Full Blood Count – especially where excessive alcohol use is suspected, to look at the Mean Corpuscular Volume (raised). Liver Function Tests will assist monitoring of liver disease where there is hepatitis and/or alcohol use. Gamma glutamyl transferase may be useful in those who deny drinking, as a concrete marker to show them at consultation. Consider checking thyroid function where there is mood instability with clinical signs and symptoms of thyroid disease.

Patients should be offered testing for Hepatitis B and C and HIV where appropriate, especially in intravenous drug users. There are also transmission risks from snorting cocaine, inadequate sterilisation procedures in overseas countries, tattooing in substandard conditions and sexual health risks, as these can be forgotten when focusing on drug-related transmission.

Other investigations

Electrocardiogram (ECG)

When the methadone dose is at a level of 100 mL or above an ECG is recommended to specifically look at the QTc interval or at a lower dose where there are other risk factors for a prolonged QTc interval (e.g. the patient is being prescribed erythromycin or risperidone). Also remind the patient of the sudden cardiac risks that cocaine poses, along with the risk of seizures and other neurological conditions, including persistent tics. A patient may have multiple cardiac risk factors in addition to methadone.

Chest X-ray

A chest X-ray may be required if there are signs of active TB or pneumonia.

Echocardiogram

An echocardiogram is required if there are signs of heart failure or a new murmur.

Management

After an initial assessment, GPs can refer the patient to the local specialist drug service. Usually there are locally agreed shared care guidelines, which involve joint working between the GP and a drug worker. GPs with a special interest in substance misuse may wish to take more responsibility for prescribing substitute medication.

Opioid dependence: maintenance and detoxification

The options of achieving abstinence from opioids, maintenance on oral opioids and harm reduction interventions should be discussed. Both methadone and buprenorphine are effective for opioid maintenance and detoxification. There is good evidence that treatment can reduce the risk of harm from blood-borne viruses, of offending behaviour and of accidental overdoses. The principles of treatment are to help the person achieve more control over drug use, improve physical and mental health, and improve social functioning. Maintenance should always be accompanied by discussion about dose changes, perhaps at three-monthly reviews. Drug prescribing should not be undertaken alone – social and psychological support should also be offered (see Box 4.1).

Box 4.1 Psychological interventions for drug misuse

1. Brief interventions
    - Used opportunistically for people not in contact with drug services (e.g. primary care). Include motivational interviewing and provision of information on reducing risk of blood borne viruses
    - Self-help groups: Narcotics Anonymous and Cocaine Anonymous (based on 12 steps principles)
2. Formal interventions – as suggested in the NICE guidelines (2007)
    - Contingency management: this involves offering incentives to reward positive behaviour such as remaining abstinent. Incentives include financial rewards, vouchers and privileges. Rewards for progress in treatment have always been available, e.g. reduced frequency of chemist visits. Payment for progress remains highly controversial.
    - Behavioural couples therapy
    - Cognitive behavioural therapy: for treatment of comorbid depression and anxiety disorders

Supervised consumption reduces the risk of overdose and diversion of controlled drugs. It is undertaken by the pharmacy dispensing the prescription. Good communication between the prescriber and the pharmacist is essential in ensuring that the patient receives the correct dose and any concerns are reported back to the prescriber. Most new patients are required to take their daily dose under direct supervision of a professional for at least three months. Most patients are stabilised on methadone at a dose of 60–120 mg. For those wishing to undergo detoxification, the dose of methadone (or buprenorphine) can be reduced gradually, over weeks or months depending on the individual. However, there is a high relapse rate, especially in the absence of social and psychological support. The drug used to stabilise the patient can also be used for detoxification, but if on a methadone prescription then buprenorphine can be considered once the dose is down to about 30 mg methadone 1 mg/1 mL mixture daily. Detoxification is usually undertaken in the community but may need to take place within a residential setting in some circumstances where community detoxification has not succeeded. Residential treatment should not be taken lightly, is expensive, and should be followed by either residential or community rehabilitation. The impulsive nature of addiction can lead people to desire a quick solution, without fully understanding the hard work that is required on their part for detoxification to succeed.

Relapse prevention

Naltrexone is an opioid antagonist used to help patients remain abstinent. It reduces the positive experience associated with use of opiates. It should be used alongside psychological interventions. Naltrexone is an opioid blocker but has also been used in the context of alcohol. It requires 7–10 days of abstinence from opioids, otherwise severe withdrawal will be precipitated. A discussion should be held with the patient about the risk of accidental overdose following loss of tolerance in abstinence. Naltrexone is also available in the private sector as an implant. It is a medication that should be prescribed by doctors familiar with managing substance misuse or with advice from experienced colleagues to ensure the best outcomes.

Alcohol dependence: detoxification

This can be performed in the community with the support of the primary care team or community mental health team and specialist drug services. Inpatient treatment is recommended for patients at risk of suicide, those with inadequate social support or history of withdrawal seizures. A reducing regime of chlordiazepoxide or diazepam (a benzodiazepine) is administered to reduce withdrawal symptoms, and thiamine and multivitamins reduce the risk of Wernicke's encephalopathy. Oxazepam is the benzodiazepine of choice where there is significant liver failure. A history of withdrawal seizures should only exclude community detoxification where the history is confirmed. People may have had withdrawal seizures when they went into prison and their alcohol withdrawal was not noted or they suddenly stopped drinking in the community, rather than a well-planned detoxification over 7 to 10 days. Repeated requests for serial alcohol detoxification in the same individual should be carefully considered due to the risk of lowering the seizure threshold. Acamprosate can be considered towards the end of the detoxification to reduce craving.

Alcohol dependence: relapse prevention

Pharmacological interventions (see Box 4.2) should be used in conjunction with psychosocial interventions such as self-help groups (Alcoholics Anonymous) and cognitive behavioural therapy.

Box 4.2 Drug treatments for maintaining abstinence from alcohol

1. Disulfiram (antabuse)
    -   Inhibits aldehyde dehydrogenase, which results in an accumulation of acetaldehyde if alcohol is consumed. This causes an unpleasant reaction (flushing, headaches, palpitations, nausea and vomiting) and therefore acts as a deterrent. Use is restricted to people who are motivated and can be supervised (e.g. by partner). Hepatotoxicity is a rare complication.
2. Acamprosate
    -   Reduces the intensity of, and response to cues and triggers of drinking.

Prescribing for benzodiazepine misuse and dependence

This is a challenging area for many prescribers; benzodiazepines are incredibly useful medications when used with caution. Unfortunately, dependence can be very difficult to treat. Patients are generally reluctant to have the dose of their benzodiazepine reduced.

Urine testing for benzodiazepines is necessary before prescribing for addiction but should not be based on one test, due to the long half-life. A prescribing contract is advised from the start of prescribing. If initiating a new prescription and an opioid substitute, waiting 4–12 weeks to stabilise the initial opioid substitute prescription is recommended. As a rough rule of thumb reduction can take place over the same number of months as the years they have been addicted, i.e. a 15 year addiction could be managed by detoxification over 15 months. Rarely, low-dose diazepam long-term may be acceptable weighed against other risks (e.g. returning to alcohol dependence). The advice is generally to convert other benzodiazepines to their diazepam equivalent using Table 4.1. However, if a plan can be made on their initial benzodiazepine medication (e.g. clonazepam) and this is the patient's choice then follow that option. The benefit of using diazepam is predominantly the low-dose tablet formulations that can be used for reduction.

Diazepam prescribing contract

The document in Box 4.3 records an agreement reached between the client and the prescriber/service regarding the regime for the prescription of diazepam.

Table 4.1 Approximate dose equivalents between diazepam and other benzodiazepines (from Department of Health, 2007).

Drug	Approximate dose equivalents
Diazepam	5 mg
Chlordiazepoxide	15 mg
Lorazepam	500 micrograms
Nitrazepam	5 mg
Oxazepam	15 mg
Temazepam	10 mg

Box 4.3 An example of a diazepam prescribing contract

We agreed that [enter name of service] will prescribe diazepam for the client to treat benzodiazepine dependency. We noted that there is little evidence to suggest that long-term substitute prescribing of benzodiazepines reduces the harm associated with benzodiazepine misuse and that there is increasing evidence that long-term prescribing may cause harm. Current guidelines advise that such prescriptions should therefore gradually reduce to zero. We therefore agreed that we will prescribe a gradually reducing dose of diazepam.

We noted that sometimes a client may feel that they can not cope with reductions in their benzodiazepine dose due to external circumstances. However, in these cases, it is clinically appropriate to continue the reduction at the pre-agreed rate as this feeling of reliance is a symptom of the benzodiazepine dependency that is being treated.

We agreed that the prescription of diazepam should commence at a dose of [X] mg daily on [X]. This dose will continue until [X] and then start reducing at a rate of [X] mg every [X] weeks until a dose of [X] mg is reached when the regime will be reviewed.

Client:
Signature:
Date:
Doctor:
Signature:
Date:
Key worker:
Signature:
Date:

DVLA issues

It is the duty of the patient to inform the DVLA if they hold a driving licence and the medication they are on, or the drugs or alcohol they use, are such that they should inform the DVLA. If they fail to do so then it is the duty of the doctor to inform the patient that the doctor has to tell the DVLA. The patient does need to know that there will then be close scrutiny by the DVLA over a significant period of time and they may have their licence withdrawn temporarily or permanently (see http://www.dvla.gov.uk/medical/ataglance.aspx). Box 4.4 is a notice that may be useful to have in your surgery.

Box 4.4 Notifying the DVLA

NOTICE TO ALL CLIENTS
Please note:

If you hold a driving licence, you are obliged by law to inform the DVLA about your substance misuse problems and any treatment you may be receiving. The DVLA may request a report from your doctor before deciding whether to allow you to drive, usually under certain conditions, or whether to temporarily suspend your licence. Failure to inform the DVLA will invalidate the insurance on any vehicle you drive and may be considered a criminal offence.

If you choose to tell a health professional that you hold a driving licence, they will then be legally obliged to inform the DVLA if they are aware that you have not done so yourself.

Prescribing in primary care

In the field of addictions one of the most problematic issues is the attitude of healthcare professionals towards individuals who misuse substances. This is clearly against the expectations of any of the professional bodies; the GMC states that it is unethical to withhold treatment on the basis of prejudice towards the aetiology of the condition. Many GPs are inclined to claim a lack of knowledge or training when dealing with patients with drug addictions and perhaps a fear of prescribing wrongly, or insufficiently, both to reduce harm and misuse of illegal substances.

In England treatment of drug users for their addiction to opioids is managed by the local enhanced schemes funded by the primary care trusts; however, all GPs are expected to be able to assess patients presenting with drug addiction, provide medical care and refer to drug and alcohol services if required.

GPs need to act in a completely non-judgemental way. Patients need to feel that they can discuss such issues with their GPs without prejudice. As addiction is a chronic, relapsing condition for a large group of patients, then the therapeutic, long-term relationship with a GP is incredibly powerful in facilitating the recovery process. Many of these patients will have had various damaging relationships in their lives, so to have a long-term, positive relationship with a professional can be very therapeutic. These patients need to normalise their behaviours in accessing health care rather than being the exception. It is possible to make a significant impact on local communities by addressing drug misuse and the criminality associated with it, and in time by reducing episodes of admission to hospital with addiction-related illnesses such as DVTs, cellulitis and endocarditis.

In the absence of insight by GPs into less than satisfactory professional behaviour, the provision of a fair and equitable health service for this exceptionally needy population, cannot be a reality. To help improve the knowledge, skills and attitudes of doctors there is now an undergraduate medical curriculum for addictions.

The three aims of the curriculum are:

- Students should be able to recognise, assess and understand the management of substance misuse and associated health and social problems and contribute to the prevention of addiction.
- Students should be aware of the effects of their own substance misuse on their own behaviour and health and on their professional practice and conduct.
- Students' education and training should challenge the stigma and discrimination that are often experienced by people with addiction problems.

The goal is to map addictions against all the disciplines taught in undergraduate medical education, as problems relating to drug and alcohol use appear in every medical specialty and are commonplace. To ignore the issue is to limit the scope of assessment and differential diagnoses and therefore limits the quality of patient care.

Key points

- Never assume; always screen for substance misuse regardless of age or cultural background.
- Never prescribe opioid substitute medication without urine confirmation of opioid use and a clinical presentation supporting dependence.
- Be aware of the local statutory and voluntary sector services available to your patients.
- Physical comorbidity is common in drug and alcohol use and may be masked by substances; always consider organic differentials to a presentation of intoxication.
- Always refer to your local GPwSI colleagues or NHS drug service medical colleagues for advice as and when required.

Further reading and bibliography

Department of Health (England) and the devolved administrations (2007) *Drug Misuse and Dependence: UK Guidelines on Clinical Management.* Department of Health (England), the Scottish Government, Welsh Assembly Government and Northern Ireland Executive. http://www.nta.nhs.uk/areas/clinical_guidance/clinical_guidelines/docs/clinical_guidelines_2007.pdf

NICE (2007) *Drug Misuse: Psychosocial Interventions.* Clinical Guidelines CG 51. National Institute for Health and Clinical Excellence. http://guidance.nice.org.uk/CG51.

NICE (2007). *Drug Misuse: Opioid Detoxification.* Clinical guidelines CG52. National Institute for Health and Clinical Excellence. http://guidance.nice.org.uk/CG52.

Useful websites

http://www.smmgp.org.uk/: a resource for GPs with training and education information, including guidelines on methadone and buprenorphine prescribing and management of cocaine users in primary care.

http://www.talktofrank.com/ incorporates a phone line (0800 77 66 00) and a website. FRANK provides free, confidential drugs information and advice 24 hours a day.

CHAPTER 5

Eating disorders

Adrienne Key and Michael Harding

Case history

A 19-year-old female presents to her GP with concerns about her menstruation. For the past four months she has not had her period, which was previously regular. She admits to having problems at home, including a difficult relationship with her mother, and is struggling to keep up with her course at college. The GP notices that she is very thin and has calluses on her knuckles. After further questioning she admits that she had been trying to lose weight as she believes that she is fat. She has been restricting her daily calorie intake to 1000 calories, and has been exercising vigorously and vomiting in order to lose weight. Her GP examines her and she is found to have a BMI of 16. She wishes to lose weight further and denies the seriousness of her condition. She is reluctant to seek treatment. The GP therefore arranges further appointments to monitor her weight and blood tests and continues to provide support. She eventually agrees to a referral to her local community mental health team.

Introduction

Eating disorders are mental illnesses characterised by a preoccupation with the control of weight, shape or food leading to extreme or chaotic eating behaviour. They are associated with specific psychological attitudes or beliefs and highly significant psychological and physical morbidity and mortality. They have been recognised as increasingly prevalent and disabling. This rapid rise may reflect better detection in addition to a true increase in incidence. Despite this it is estimated that many eating disorders go undetected, including half the cases of anorexia nervosa and a greater number of bulimic or atypical disorders. Prevalence and incidence vary according to the study examined but the most conservative estimate for anorexia nervosa is 0.3% of the population and for bulimia nervosa is 1% (Hoek, 2006). Anorexia and bulimia are subgroups of a much larger group of eating disorders, clinically very similar but which do not meet precise criteria (Hoek, 2006). These atypical eating disorders are associated with equal morbidity and mortality as anorexia and bulimia and probably double the number of eating disorders in the population (Hoek, 2006). Ninety per cent of eating disorders occur in women aged 15–25 in Western society, but increasing numbers of cases are being recognised across the age range and in men.

Aetiology of eating disorders

Research has now clearly demonstrated that the causes of eating disorders are multifactorial, some predisposing an individual to illness, others acting as a trigger or maintaining factor.

Biological factors

Biological factors are thought to be genetically mediated. The inherited liability probably involves relevant personality traits such as perfectionism, obsessionality and high anxiety levels. These probably predispose to difficulties in modulating/maintaining a healthy self-esteem or lead to a vulnerability to societal dieting pressure. Obsessionality and perfectionism are also associated with the adoption of ascetic behaviours. Recent research has concentrated on the brain's response to starvation/dieting, including brain blood flow changes in areas associated with emotions and body image and alterations in neurotransmitters in individuals with eating disorders. Theories suggest that when a biologically vulnerable individual diets or loses weight, these biological changes occur, creating the eating disorder. Starvation also produces experiences of low or labile moods, emotional blunting, obsessional thinking and preoccupation with food.

Psychological factors

Individuals with low self-esteem are vulnerable to eating disorders. Psychological factors common to sufferers include those associated with the development of low self-esteem and include difficult relationships, family dysfunction, traumatic events, life events, teasing and bullying (particularly about weight). Life events trigger eating problems, perhaps through causing low mood or self-doubt, leading to dieting or weight loss. Adolescence is associated with the development of anorexia nervosa and it is thought that premorbid personality traits, such as perfectionism and low self-esteem, make negotiating this time of change too difficult.

Social factors

Eating disorders are associated with a western culture or one undergoing a rapid change towards a western ideal. This has led to many hypotheses about the social factors important in eating disorders including the over-valuation of the thin body ideal. The impact of media in promoting thinness or physical perfection is believed to promote increasing levels of body dissatisfaction and hence more extreme methods of weight control.

History

Patients with eating disorders frequently present asking for help, but can also present atypically, and therefore GPs need to be vigilant to their presence. Sufferers may not recognise their eating disorder as an illness or as problematic, while others feel guilt and shame, making accessing appropriate help difficult. NICE (2004) guidelines (Box 5.1) highlight some at-risk groups where the clinician's index of suspicion should be raised. A screening instrument such as

---

Box 5.1 NICE guidelines for at risk groups

Target groups for screening

- Women with low BMI
- Type 1 diabetes
- GI problems, starvation symptoms (raised LFTs, anaemia)
- Repeated vomiting (low potassium)
- Children with poor growth
- Normal weight people consulting with weight concerns
- Menstrual disturbance, infertility

Box 5.2 The SCOFF questionnaire

- Do you make yourself **S**ick because you feel uncomfortably full?
- Do you worry you have lost **C**ontrol over how much you eat?
- Have you recently lost more than **O**ne stone in a 3 month period?
- Do you believe yourself to be **F**at when others say you are too thin?
- Would you say that **F**ood dominates your life?

One point for every 'Yes'; a score of 2 indicates a likely case of an eating disorder (Morgan *et al.*, 1999).

SCOFF (Box 5.2) may allow early detection (Morgan *et al.*, 1999). Frequently carers present requesting support for young people whose insight is still limited. The GP's approach must be supportive and collaborative (a motivational stance), engaging the patient both in revealing the problem and motivating them towards help (Treasure and Schmidt, 2008). It may take the patient two or more appointments before they reveal the nature and extent of their worries.

Throughout the assessment the clinician should enable the patient to explore the negative effects of the eating disorder, and why they now choose to seek help or finally allow others to know of its existence. The clinician should convey their understanding of the illness, its biological underpinnings and how confusing patients find their myriad of conflicting emotions. Ambivalence to treatment is always present and will remain for a long time, this is to be expected by both clinician and patient. The clinician, by using a motivational stance, helps the patient see ambivalence and choose to move towards treatment by their own volition and motivation. The clinician must establish a diagnosis, assess the level of risk and then jointly decide on a treatment path.

Step 1: Assessment

A detailed description of the current problem should be obtained using questions that cover the different domains of the DSM-IV diagnoses (Box 5.3), and physical, psychological and social complications of the illnesses. These can be distilled down into a more manageable list for example in Box 5.4! Always briefly enquire about school/employment, social life, peer group, relationships and family as eating disorders are associated with high levels of dysfunction, low quality of life, poor relationships and social support networks. This can help the patient to gather insight into how the disorder is affecting all aspects of her life.

Box 5.3 DSM-IV criteria for eating disorders (DSM-IV, 1994)

307.1 Anorexia nervosa

A. Refusal to maintain body weight at or above a minimally normal weight for age and height (body weight less than 85% of that expected or body mass index of 17.5 and below.

B. Intense fear of gaining weight or becoming fat, even though underweight.

C. Disturbance in the way in which one's body weight or shape is experienced, undue influence of body shape or weight on self-evaluation, or denial of the seriousness of the current low body weight.

D. In postmenarcheal females, amenorrhea, i.e. the absence of at least three consecutive menstrual cycles.

Subtypes: Restricting type and binge-eating/purging type – depending on whether person has regularly engaged in binge eating or purging behaviour (i.e. self-induced vomiting or the misuse of laxatives, diuretics or enemas).

307.51 Bulimia nervosa

A. Recurrent episodes of binge eating. An episode of binge eating is characterised by both of the following:

  (1) Eating, in a discrete period of time (e.g. within a 2-hour period), an amount of food that is definitely larger than most people would eat during a similar period of time and under similar circumstances.

  (2) A sense of lack of control over eating during the episode (e.g. a feeling that one cannot stop eating or control what or how much one is eating).

B. Recurrent inappropriate compensatory behaviour in order to prevent weight gain, such as self-induced vomiting, misuse of laxatives, diuretics, enemas, or other medications, fasting or excessive exercise.

C. The binge eating and compensatory behaviours both occur on average at least twice a week for 3 months.

D. Self-evaluation is unduly influenced by body shape and weight.

E. The disturbance does not occur exclusively during episodes of anorexia nervosa.

Subtypes: Purging type and non purging type – depending on regular use of purging behaviours or other behaviours (e.g. fasting/exercise)

307.50 Eating Disorder Not Otherwise Specified (EDNOS)

The EDNOS category is for disorders of eating that do not meet the full criteria for any specific eating disorder.

Box 5.4 Assessment questions

1. Eating and behaviours
   - What do you eat on an average day?
   - What foods do you avoid?
   - Do you ever go most of the day without food?
   - Do you ever vomit, exercise, take laxatives or diuretics? If so when and how much?
   - Do you ever feel you lose control or binge? How often?
   - If I met you 6 months/3 months/1 month ago how different was your weight?
   - What do you weigh?/How tall are you?
2. Psychological attitudes
   - How do you feel about your weight? What weight would you like to be?
   - How would you feel if you gained half a stone?
   - How much of the day are you burdened by thoughts of food, weight or your body shape?
   - Do you feel down or guilty or suicidal?
3. Physical effects
   - When was your last period?
   - How are you sleeping?
   - Have you felt dizzy when standing lately?
   - Are you more sensitive to the cold?
   - Are your bowels upset or does your stomach hurt?
   - Are you feeling weak or finding it harder to exercise now?
4. Impact on life
   - Are you still going out/socialising like you used to?
   - Do you feel seeing people is 'just too much' now?
   - Can you still concentrate at school/work? Are you still going?
   - How are your friends/partner/family? Has anything changed lately between you?
   - Are you feeling on your own with this?

If the child is premenarchal then questions should target any possible growth retardation, pubertal delay or arrest as this is more commonly the clinical picture rather than gross weight loss.

Comorbid conditions such as depression, anxiety, obsessive compulsive disorder, alcohol, drug misuse (including diet pills) and self-harm maybe present and alter the level of risk (risk assessment below). The clinician must also understand why and when the patient developed an eating disorder. What predisposing vulnerabilities does the patient demonstrate and what precipitating factors were relevant? This importantly enables the GP to educate the patient about the nature of their illness particularly the biological component, thus improving insight. Most patients are very confused about what is happening to them, realising eating disorders are definable illnesses and understood by their GP helps move them to a position of accepting help.

Examination

Eating disorders, particularly anorexia nervosa, are associated with six times the standardised mortality rate. Physical complications include premature death by cardiovascular complications, infection or organ failure. Purging behaviours cause hypokalaemia and cardiac arrhythmias, but low body weight is also a factor. Low oestrogen (or testosterone in men) and high levels of stress hormones produced by chaotic eating and low weight cause osteoporosis and infertility. The miscarriage rate doubles and the perinatal mortality is six times the normal. In adolescents the poor nutrition associated with eating disorders leads to pubertal delay or arrest, growth retardation and short stature and severe osteoporosis. Physical assessment is vital!

Step 2: The physical examination

The aim of the physical examination is to determine the effects of starvation in underweight patients. The NICE guidelines recommend that, as a minimum, GPs should check the patient's height, weight and Body Mass Index (weight (kg)/height (metres)^2, and for children under the age of 18 the use of growth centile charts is recommended. A BMI of 18.5–25 is normal. In children, data about previous developmental stage, growth and puberty reached prior to the illness give a more dynamic picture. This leads to an understanding of the presence and extent of any growth retardation, pubertal delay or arrest or reduction of peak bone mass caused by the eating disorder. This should be included in addition to the examination. The patient's pulse and blood pressure should also be checked.

Further examination may be required if there are concerns about physical instability (see Table 5.1).

For someone who is purging, the GP must be vigilant for signs of dehydration, postural hypotension, arrthymias, hypokalaemia and hyponatraemia. The squat test is a useful test as it is sensitive to falling weight arising from muscle

Table 5.1 Physical examination for a patient with an eating disorder.

Systems review	Examination
Cardiovascular	Blood pressure, pulse, heart sounds, peripheral perfusion (looking for postural and resting hypotension, bradycardia, palpitations, arrthymias, poor peripheral perfusion)
Skin and hair	Lanugo hair, emaciation, dry skin, cyanosis, jaundice, head hair loss, swollen parotid glands (vomiting) or calluses on the hand knuckles (Russell's sign due to vomiting using fingers down the throat), self-mutilation
Musculoskeletal	Myopathy of limb girdle muscles, general weakness, (squat test), fractures due to osteopenia/osteoporosis, tooth decay due to enamel loss (secondary to vomiting)
Metabolic	Liver problems, hypothermia, dehydration, (tests to establish hypoglycaemia, hypokalaemia, hyponatraemia)
Renal	Tests to establish renal failure
CNS	Starvation induced poor concentration, poor alertness or general poor understanding, tetany, fits, evidence of drug misuse (particularly caffeine, slimming pills/amphetamines)
Other	Weigh and height your patient!

loss and can be detected through weekly tests. The patient squats all the way down to the floor and attempts to stand up without using his or her hands for leverage:

- Score of 0: Unable to stand up.
- Score of 1: Able to stand up only by using hands to pull up.
- Score of 2: Able to stand up without using hands, but with noticeable difficulty.
- Score of 3: Able to stand up without difficulty.

If patient scores 0 or 1 or deteriorates over the week this indicates significant muscle loss and thus physical deterioration due to starvation.

Investigations

Step 3: Investigations

A basic blood screen of urea and electrolytes, liver function tests with calcium and phosphate and full blood count are required. An electrocardiogram should be considered, particularly if BMI is less than 15, if there are electrolyte abnormalities, cardiac compromise or bradycardia (Table 5.2). A urinary drug screen may also be indicated from the history. A pelvic ultrasound or DEXA bone scan to identify osteoporosis may be useful later in treatment, but is usually undertaken in secondary care.

Table 5.2 Essential tests for a patient with an eating disorder (http://www. eatingresearch.com/).

Investigation	Comments
1. Urea and electrolytes	Check in all patients, particularly those with purging behaviours (vomiting, laxative or diuretic abuse). The most common finding is low potassium
2. Liver function tests	Raised levels are very common in starvation. Bilirubin level is only rarely elevated.
3. Creatine kinase	Increase shows muscle is being used as a source of energy. CK is mostly skeletal although the cardiac fraction is also sometimes elevated, indicating probable cardiac damage
4. Haematology, full blood count	Bone marrow suppression secondary to starvation may be present
5. Electrocardiograph (ECG)	Important in all patients but also for any patient who has lost weight rapidly or who demonstrates cardiovascular abnormalities on examination. Bradycardia is common (< 55/min). The most important abnormalities to rule out are arrthymias and conduction problems, indicated by a prolonged (> 420 ms) corrected QT interval

Management and discussion

Step 4: Assessment of risk

The assessment of risk is established to inform both the clinician and patient of how to proceed. A detailed explanation of results to the patient is vital. Medical and psychological risk are equally important and include the assessment of insight/capacity and motivation for treatment.

Medical/physical risk

The results of the physical examination and investigations give an indication of the level of medical risk (Table 5.3). High risk (alert) indicates immediate referral to secondary or specialist eating disorder services. Moderate risk (concern) indicates weekly monitoring with referral to secondary or specialist eating disorder services. Low risk indicates treatment options within primary care with monitoring.

Psychological risk

High risk includes those who are a suicide risk but also patients with comorbid conditions, particularly addictions, depression and self-harm. Assessment will include why has the patent presented now? What has changed recently? Has self-harm started or changed?

When to seek referral or discussion

Step 5: Assess capacity and insight

Eating disorders are associated with high levels of guilt, shame and extremely painful experiences of self-hatred and self-consciousness. Anorexia is also frequently not viewed by the sufferer as an illness but rather a vital necessity for self-worth. So a patient may not wish for any intervention, or may be a child brought by concerned parents or friend/carers consulting the GP.

Table 5.3 Physical risk assessment.

System	Test	Concern	Alert
Nutrition	BMI	<14	<12
	Weight loss/week	> 0.5 kg	> 1.0 kg
Circulation	Systolic BP	< 90	< 80
	Diastolic BP	< 70	< 60
	Postural drop	> 10	> 20
	Pulse rate	< 50	< 40
Squat test	Score 2		
	Score 1	++	
	Score 0		++
Temperature		< 35 °C	< 34.5 °C
FBC	WCC	< 4.0	< 2.0
	Hb	< 11	< 9
	Platelets	< 130	< 110
U&Es	K^+	< 3.5	< 3.0
	Na^+	< 135	< 130
	PO^{4-}	0.5–0.8	< 0.5
	Urea	> 7	> 10
Liver	Bilirubin	> 20	> 40
	AST	> 40	> 80
	ALT	> 45	> 90
ECG	Pulse rate	< 50	< 40
	Corrected QT (QTC)		> 450 ms
	Arrythmias		++

Concern = regular review with referral to ED or secondary services
Alert = immediate urgent referral to ED or secondary services

The patient may be obviously underweight but refusing help. Risk assessment will therefore include assessment of capacity and may require the use of the Mental Heath Act. If capacity or insight is compromised or if risk is high the GP should seek support at this stage with the relevant psychiatric counterpart (Child and Adolescent Mental Health Services (CAMHS), Community Mental Health Services (CMHS) or Eating Disorder Services (EDS)) to discuss joint assessment or referral. All children with eating disorders should be discussed with secondary services and most adults with anorexia nervosa will require specialist intervention.

Treatment in primary care

Step 6: Treatment aims

For adults when risk is low, treatment can commence in primary care. The GP's role is to:

- Continue medical monitoring and charting (maybe weekly)
- Establish a therapeutic relationship
- Focus on regular eating; dietitian if available
- Educate about physical consequences of weight-reducing behaviours
- Support accessing help (self-help books, Beat website, seeing a therapist)

Self-help books have proven worth (Box 5.5). They allow the patient to gather information at their own pace or work jointly with the GP or counsellor. NICE guidelines (2004) also indicate the use of fluoxetine 60 mg for bulimia. The GP should also promote self-help by recommending the Beat website. Beat is the leading charity in the UK for all types of eating disorders and offer a plethora of expert information, online support and guidance as well as actual groups for sufferers and carers in the community.

Box 5.5 Recommended self-help resources

Books

Overcoming Binge Eating by Dr Christopher Fairburn
Getting Better Bite by Bite by Ulrike Schmidt and Janet Treasure
Anorexia Nervosa. A survival Guide for Sufferers and Those Caring for Someone with an Eating Disorder by Janet Treasure
Skills-based Learning in Caring for a Loved One with an Eating Disorder: The new Maudsley Method, by J. Treasure, G. Smith and A. Crane

Website
Beat (formerly the Eating Disorders Association): http://www.b-eat.co.uk/.

A specific form of CBT is recommended for patients with bulimia and binge eating disorders not responding to the above interventions (CBT-BN for 16–20 sessions), and can be delivered by trained therapists in primary care. There is evidence that CBT-BN reduces the frequency of binge eating and purging behaviours (NICE, 2004). It specifically looks at eating habits and attitudes. An alternative form of therapy, Interpersonal Psychotherapy (IPT), concentrates on interpersonal issues and not food/behaviours. The number of sessions required can be more and results take longer to achieve, but it is equally as effective as CBT-BN for bulimic disorders. Some patients clearly prefer this approach from the outset, but it should also be considered if patients find the CBT ineffective after the first six sessions. It is vital that treatment works constantly to address and promote motivation in the patient through supporting them and recognising that if a specific form of treatment does not help a patient this does not make the illness 'untreatable' – it is merely not working for that individual and other approaches should be sought. This is the norm in anorexia nervosa or anorectic type illnesses particularly because of the ever-present ambivalence and fear of treatment the patient may experience. Failure to acknowledge this by the clinicians will leave the patient feeling misunderstood, causing disengagement and treatment failure. There are treatment trials in anorexia nervosa looking at the use of cognitive models (Maudsley model and the Oxford group) and IPT which are producing encouraging results for patients whose insight has grown and who have reached the stage of moving forward, but these are probably currently only available in secondary services and above.

For the GP treating a patient with anorexia nervosa in primary care, physical monitoring may have to be a weekly occurrence, especially in those who progress in weight gain. This is to avoid 'refeeding syndrome' caused by micronutrient deficiencies, particularly phosphate, brought about by rapid refeeding and anabolic processes within a starved and depleted body. Refeeding syndrome can be detected by a dropping phosphate level and worsening liver function tests. A full syndrome, which is very rare, can lead to cardiovascular collapse, coma or death. If the patient is slowly refed, starting them on under 1000 kcal a day and only moving up slowly to 1500 kcal over the first 10 days in conjunction with a good quality multivitamin mineral preparation (forceval 1 cap daily), refeeding syndrome can be avoided.

Treatment in secondary and specialist care

Children with eating disorders require physical monitoring, looking at their developmental stage and progression as well as current physical risk, in conjunction with specialist family work. For these reasons referral onto CAMHS or specialist eating disorder services is recommended for outpatient treatment. Family interventions in the form of assessment, participation in treatment, formal family work and carers support/groups are central to treatment for all children – research has clearly demonstrated this and NICE guidelines recommend it. There is no evidence to suggest that conjoint family therapy (patient and family see therapist together) is more or less superior to separate family therapy (patient and family see therapist separately). Research has also explored the use of 'multi-family therapy' which has produced very encouraging results. Families are seen together as a large group for an intensive period of therapy. The supportive nature of this type of approach has empowered parents/carers and enabled them to help their member with anorexia more effectively. When outpatient treatment fails, day or inpatient treatment can be considered. The institution to which the youngster is admitted should be age-appropriate, with expertise in treating eating disorders, and should offer educational support.

Adults with eating disorders are also mainly treated as outpatients. Those with bulimia and life-threatening purging or severely self-damaging behaviour may require admission. The majority of patients admitted as day or inpatients have anorexia nervosa and are deemed 'high risk' (see above) or have not progressed as outpatients. Adult eating disorder units offer comprehensive therapies with a range of individual, group and practical approaches to meet the physical, social and psychological needs of patients. Dietary advice and a prescribed pattern of eating are standard, alongside expected weight gain of 0.5 kg a week and physical monitoring. There is very little evidence supporting the use of one form of individual psychological therapy over another.

When the illness is life-threatening and the patient lacks the insight into their anorexia, detention under the Mental Health Act and nasogastric feeding may be necessary. These are a last resort to save life. When assisted feeding is required it should only be under the guidance of an eating disorder specialist (NICE, 2004). Control should be restored to the patient as rapidly as possible to enable restoration of the autonomy necessary for full recovery, but only if stability and progression have been established.

Prognosis

The mean crude mortality of anorexia nervosa is 5%. Full recovery occurs in about half the surviving patients, with a third showing some improvement and a fifth following a chronic course (Steinhausen, 2002). Predictors of poor outcome in patients with anorexia nervosa include low BMI at presentation, older age (over 20 years), bulimic subtype, premorbid personality difficulties, body image disturbance and family disturbance (NICE, 2004). In patients with bulimia nervosa, predictors of poor outcome include features of borderline personality disorder, substance misuse and higher levels of binge-eating and purging (NICE, 2004).

Conclusions

Eating disorders can be severe and disabling mental illnesses that frequently elude detection. If the GP is vigilant to their presence then the patient can be helped and many of the long-term complications may be avoided. The GP's task is to diagnose, assess risk and motivate the patient towards the start of help. Many patients can be successfully treated in primary care and outpatients; inpatient treatment is a last resort.

Key points

- Be vigilant to the presence of an eating disorder, particularly in high-risk groups.
- Engage the patient using a motivational approach at all times.
- Assessment includes physical, psychological and social parameters. High risk can be defined through specific criteria.
- Physical monitoring of the patient should continue throughout treatment.
- Seek advice and possible referral for all children and adolescents with eating disorders and those with anorexia nervosa at lower weights.
- Treatment includes the use of self-help books and the Beat website.

Further reading and bibliography

Hoek, H. W. (2006) Incidence, prevalence and mortality of anorexia and other eating disorders. *Current Opinion in Psychiatry*, **19**, 389–94.

Morgan, J. F., Reid, F. and Lacey, J. H. (1999) The SCOFF questionnaire: assessment of a new screening tool for eating disorders. *British Medical Journal*, **319**, 1467–8.

NICE (2004) *Eating Disorders: Core Interventions in the Management of Anorexia Nervosa, Bulimia Nervosa and Related Eating Disorders.* Clinical guidelines CG9. National Institute for Health and Clinical Excellence. http://guidance.nice.org.uk/CG9.

Steinhausen, H. C. (2002) The outcome of anorexia nervosa in the 20th century. *American Journal of Psychiatry*, **159**, 1284–93.

Treasure, J. and Schmidt, U. (2008) Motivational interviewing in eating disorders. In: *Motivational Interviewing and the Promotion of Mental Health* (eds. H. Arkowitz, H. Westra, W. R. Miller and S. Rollnick), pp. 194–224. Guildford Press, New York.

Useful website

http://www.eatingresearch.com/: Information on eating disorders from the Section of Eating Disorders at the Institute of Psychiatry and the Eating Disorders Unit at the South London and Maudsley Trust.

CHAPTER 6

Organic psychiatry

Luke Solomons and Joyce Solomons

Case history

A 76-year-old lady is brought to the surgery by her husband – she has been tearful and upset for three days and her husband thinks she might be depressed. In private, she reveals to you that her husband is going to divorce her after 51 years of marriage and is having sex with a young woman at night. She also thinks he is growing vermin in the house and has seen spiders, mice and roaches on the walls and carpet. Her past medical history includes well-controlled hypertension, non-insulin-dependent diabetes mellitus managed on oral medication, and macular degeneration. Examination reveals that she is disorientated to time and place and has prominent visual hallucinations without an auditory component and paranoid delusions. A urine dipstick reveals blood and protein in her urine and a subsequent culture reveals heavy growth of *E. coli*.

A course of trimethoprim treats the urinary tract infection (UTI) and the confusion and paranoid delusions disappear, but visual hallucinations continue. She is given a trial of risperidone, but the hallucinations persist and she becomes very drowsy and stiff, so it is discontinued. An occupational therapist assesses her at home and suggests improved lighting and day centre attendance. Over time, she comes to recognise that the hallucinations are not real and is no longer distressed when she experiences them.

Introduction

Organic psychiatry encompasses disorders that arise from demonstrable abnormalities of brain structure and function. In the *Tenth Revision of the Inter-*

national Classification of Diseases and Related Health Problems (ICD-10) (World Health Organization, 1992), the term 'organic' implies that a syndrome so classified can be attributed to an independently diagnosable cerebral or systemic disease. The dysfunction may be primary, as in diseases, injuries and insults that affect the brain directly and selectively; or secondary, as in systemic diseases and disorders that attack the brain only as one of the multiple organs or systems of the body that are involved. The boundaries are blurred, however, because other psychiatric disorders like schizophrenia have some neurobiological basis; and organic mental disorders can be precipitated by psychological factors. Box 6.1 lists symptoms suggestive of an organic cause.

Box 6.1 Presentations that could imply an organic cause (in addition to psychiatric symptoms)

- Altered consciousness
- Fluctuating level of consciousness and confusion
- Memory problems
- Visual, olfactory, somatic and gustatory hallucinations (generally *not* auditory hallucinations)
- Sphincter disturbance

Classification

The ICD-10 classifies organic mental disorders from F00 to F09. This includes three major categories:

1. Delirium (F05)
2. Dementia (F00–F03)
3. Other organic syndromes – including mood disorders, anxiety, hallucinosis, delusional disorder, personality disorder (F04–F09)

Delirium

Delirium is an impairment of cognitive function that is not progressive and (most importantly) is reversible if the underlying cause is treated. Compared to the prevalence in the older adult inpatient population (up to 40%), it is rare in the community (1–2%), but it is associated with a high rate of mortality (up to 25%). People over 65 are particularly vulnerable. The terms 'acute confusional state' and 'acute organic syndrome' have been used to describe delirium in the past. It has a wide range of causes (Table 6.1).

Delirium commonly presents as acutely disturbed consciousness with disorientation in time and place, which fluctuates over the course of the day, and is typically worse in the evening (sundowning). Attention and concentration are particularly poor and there could either be agitation and restlessness or psychomotor retardation and apathy. Psychotic features and mood disturbances can present along with a marked deterioration in cognition.

Management of delirium primarily involves identifying and treating the underlying cause. Attentive care with frequent reassurance and reorientation and nursing in a quiet room avoiding sensory deprivation helps. Drug treatment is warranted only to reduce distress and exhaustion. Small doses of antipsychotics such as haloperidol given regularly are preferred. Benzodiazepines can help with sleep, but will worsen confusion so should be avoided.

Table 6.1 Common causes of delirium.

Cause	Example
Drug intoxication or withdrawal	Alcohol, anticholinergics, sedatives, steroids, opiods, antipsychotics, antidepressants
Infection	UTI, pneumonia, septicaemia, encephalitis, meningitis, HIV infection
Metabolic causes	Dehydration, worsening chronic obstructive pulmonary disease, heart failure, uraemia, liver failure
Endocrinopathies	Hypoglycemia, diabetic ketoacidosis and hyperosmolar nonketotic syndrome (HONK), hypo/hyperthyroidism, Cushing's syndrome, hypopituitarism
Head injury	subdural haematoma, post concussional syndrome, diffuse injury
Epilepsy	Post-ictal, status epilepticus
Stroke	Intracerebral bleeds, ischaemic strokes
Tumours	Intracranial primary and secondaries, paraneoplastic syndromes
Others	Vitamin deficiencies, chronic pain, sleep disorders, constipation

Disorders of memory

Dementia is covered in Chapter 12.

Amnestic syndromes

An amnestic syndrome is defined as an abnormal mental state in which memory and learning are affected out of all proportion to other cognitive functions in an otherwise alert and responsive patient (Victor *et al.*, 1971).

The *Korsakoff syndrome* can be defined as the same but with the following phrase added: '... resulting from nutritional depletion, notably thiamine deficiency'. Many cases of the Korsakoff syndrome are diagnosed following acute Wernicke encephalopathy, involving confusion, ataxia, nystagmus and ophthalmoplegia. Confabulation is sometimes associated, but not always. Chronic alcohol abuse is the most frequent cause. A short history prior to diagnosis and prompt thiamine replacement is associated with the best prognosis. Prevalence estimates range from 0.4–2% in the population.

Transient global amnesia (TGA) is characterised by repetitive questioning, and there may be some confusion, but patients do not report any loss of personal identity. It is sometimes preceded by headache or nausea, a stressful life event, a medical procedure, intense emotion or vigorous exercise. Complete recovery is usual. Transient epileptic amnesia refers to the minority of TGA cases in whom epilepsy appears to be the underlying cause.

Psychiatric presentations of other disorders

Parkinson's disease

Psychiatric symptoms seen in Parkinson's disease include depressive illness, bradyphrenia (slowness in mental processing) and cognitive impairment. Approximately 40% of patients with Parkinson's suffer from depression and the association is well established. Management includes selective serotonin reuptake inhibitors (SSRIs) and newer antidepressants that have low anticholinergic activity. Patients with refractory depression can be referred for ECT treatment. Psychosocial support, including CBT, can be helpful.

Cognitive impairment is associated with Parkinson's disease, and correlates with the severity of the movement disorder and duration of the illness.

These patients are also especially vulnerable to delirium due to drugs or inter-current infection.

Treatment of Parkinson's disease with dopamine replacement can produce psychotic symptoms – visual hallucinations occur in 20–30%, and occasion-ally paranoid delusions. Reduction in dose is the first line of management, but if this results in unacceptable worsening of symptoms, antipsychotic medica-tion like quetiapine might be necessary. Dopamine agonist therapy has also been associated rarely with problem gambling.

Sleep disorders, including Rapid Eye Movement (REM) behaviour disor-der, are more common. Dopamine agonist therapy is linked to sleep attacks and patients must be warned not to drive if they have such episodes.

Huntington's disease

Patients present in middle life with jerky movements. This is a genetic disor-der that is autosomal dominant in its inheritance pattern. Patients can become depressed in the early stages when they have insight. Cognitive and behav-ioural decline is progressive, and mood and psychotic symptoms are common as the disease progresses, with prevalence estimates for psychiatric problems ranging from 33% to 75%. Dopaminergic blockade with antipsychotics like olanzapine might be required to suppress severe chorea, and this might help with psychotic symptoms and act as a mood stabiliser. Antidepressants are useful for depressive symptoms.

Infections

Human Immunodeficiency Virus (HIV)

HIV can cause a range of psychiatric symptoms through early invasion of the central nervous system. Emotional distress is common due to the nature of the symptoms and associated social stigma, especially in patients with previous psychological problems. HIV encephalopathy and subacute encephalitis can present, as well as HIV-associated dementia, which is due to direct effects of the virus on the brain. Immunocompromised patients are vulnerable to sec-ondary infections like toxoplasmosis or malignancy (lymphomas) that can be symptomatic. Antiretroviral therapy in itself can be associated with neuropsy-chiatric side-effects including psychosis, irritability and sleep disorders – some commonly used drugs like efavirenz are particularly implicated.

Neurosyphilis

The manifestation of the tertiary stage of infection has seen a resurgence associated with HIV. General Paralysis of the Insane (GPI) is the classically described tertiary syndrome, but symptoms can be protean – from asymptomatic neurosyphilis to florid psychosis with personality change and Tabes Dorsalis.

Encephalitis

This could be primary infection of the brain or a secondary complication of meningitis, septicaemia or brain abscess. Herpes simplex encephalitis is relatively common and can cause chronic sequelae including profound amnesia when it affects the medial temporal lobes and temporal lobe epilepsy.

Prion diseases

These neurodegenerative disorders are rare – Creutzfeldt Jakob Disease (CJD) is the most common amongst them. The interest in these diseases resulted from the description of variant CJD, linked to bovine spongiform encephalopathy (BSE). Patients can present with depressive symptoms initially, which are followed by a rapidly progressive dementia.

Brain tumours

Psychiatric manifestations of brain tumours depend on the size and location of the tumour, its rate of growth and whether or not intracranial pressure is raised. Primary tumours of the brain and meninges can be slow-growing and present with neuropsychiatric symptoms without many neurological signs (e.g. frontal gliomas). Rapidly expanding tumours can cause raised intracranial pressure with impaired concentration, impaired consciousness, drowsiness and delirium. Metastases account for 20% of intracranial neoplasms. Seizures are the most common presenting sign of a brain tumour.

Multiple sclerosis (MS)

MS can present with diverse neurological signs which reflect the distribution of demyelinating plaques. The prevalence of depression and other psychiatric problems is thought to be as high as 50% and interferon therapy for MS can worsen depressive illness. Emotional lability and uncontrollable laughing and crying can be present. Treatment with antidepressants can help. Some patients can present a decline in cognitive function and subcortical dementia.

Head injury

A number of psychiatric symptoms have been described following head injury, including emotional symptoms, personality change (particularly if there is frontal lobe damage) and serious permanent memory impairments. The duration of post-traumatic amnesia is a rough prognostic indicator of the extent of cognitive impairment.

Many patients describe symptoms after mild head injury that is grouped under post-concussional syndrome – anxiety, depression, irritability associated with headaches, poor concentration, fatigue and insomnia. The severity and duration of symptoms is variable but most cases resolve without specific intervention.

Management includes long-term multidisciplinary treatment plans with invaluable input from a clinical psychologist with behavioural and cognitive techniques and support for carers.

Cerebrovascular disease – stroke

Strokes can produce cognitive impairment depending on the site and size of the event – some specific deficits of higher functioning like dyspraxias, dysphasias and anosognosia might be hard to recognise but result in big handicaps. Small, repeated strokes and transient ischaemic attacks might sometimes take the form of a subcortical dementia, termed Binswanger's disease.

Stroke is strongly associated with depression, with estimated prevalence rates of up to 65% of patients following a stroke, and can impede rehabilitation and also present as a pseudodementia. The controversy about the location of the lesion determining the risk of depression still continues without any clear results – there is some non-replicated evidence to suggest that left hemisphere stroke is more strongly associated with depression than right hemisphere stroke. Management is by treating cautiously with antidepressants, usually SSRIs.

Stroke can also cause emotional disorders – irritability, lability of mood, apathy and, in an extreme form, catastrophic reaction (a sudden explosive outburst of rage and distress often prompted by the recognition of failing powers).

In the elderly and patients with alcohol dependence, subdural haematomas must be considered after falls. Patients can present several weeks after the incident with vague complaints like headache, dizziness, poor concentration and fluctuating consciousness. Management is surgical, which may reverse the symptoms.

Epilepsy

The paroxysmal electrical discharge in the brain causing recurrent seizures can cause various psychiatric problems – the prevalence of comorbid psychiatric symptoms is estimated to be 20–30%. Peri-ictal problems are well described.

Anxiety, irritability, emotional lability and depression can be prodromal symptoms for days before a seizure. Complex partial seizures can cause confusional states, hallucinations, mood disturbances and automatic behaviours during seizure activity. Absence seizures can cause altered awareness and automatisms. Non-convulsive status epilepticus can be misdiagnosed as dementia. Post-ictal confusional states, psychosis and mood disorders are common and often unrecognised, as is Todd's paresis (post-ictal hemiparesis, dysphasia).

Historically people with epilepsy were stigmatised, and it was thought to be a mental disorder. Until the 19th century it was thought that cognitive decline was inevitable – it has since been clearly established that relatively few people show deficits. Deficits could be due to side-effects of anti-epileptic medication, unrecognised seizures or underlying structural damage. The 'sticky, epileptic personality' was also described in the past, but has been discarded. A minority of sufferers have serious personality difficulties. Depression is more common in this population. Management is by accurate diagnosis and psychotropic drug treatment. Psychotropics might increase seizure frequency, and this must be kept in mind.

Antiepileptic medication can have psychiatric side-effects directly (e.g. vigabatrin- or topiramate-related mood disorder or psychosis), but can also have indirect effects on the mental state (e.g. drowsiness impairing academic performance, gingival hyperplasia from phenytoin causing stigma, and depression in an adolescent)

Non-epileptic seizures can be diagnostically challenging, especially if they co-exist with a seizure disorder. Identification of psychological factors causing stress and addressing them with psychosocial interventions such as cognitive behavioural therapy can help.

Charles Bonnet syndrome

Charles Bonnet syndrome is a common cause of complex visual hallucination with prevalence estimates of 10% to 15% in people with visual impairments like macular degeneration. They present with well-formed, vivid, elaborate visual hallucinations. Treatment with drugs remains unsatisfactory and increasing insight, improving lighting at home and social support may help.

Systemic illnesses

Endocrine problems

Diabetes is a chronic condition, and psychosocial problems are commonly associated. Hypothyroidism can present with depression and apathy, also with mental slowing resembling dementia. Lithium maintenance treatment for bipolar disorder can cause hypothyroidism. Hyperthyroidism can present with acute onset anxiety, agitation, irritability and occasionally manic symptoms. Patients with Cushing's disease, Addison's disease and hypopituitarism can present with low mood and apathy. Steroid therapy can cause mood symptoms and increased aggression.

Systemic lupus erythematosis

The CNS is affected in 50–75% of lupus patients and cerebral lupus can present with psychosis or mood and anxiety disorders. Subcortical infarcts can cause disturbances of cognition.

Renal problems and electrolyte imbalances

Hyponatremia can cause fatigue, lassitude, apathy and seizures – SSRI treatment in the elderly can precipitate hyponatraemia. Hypokalaemic muscle paralysis may be diagnosed as hysteria, especially in cases of familial periodic paralysis in which the hypokalaemia may be triggered by emotional stress. Depression is frequently seen in patients with end stage renal failure on haemodialysis, and uraemia can be the cause of delirium.

Sleep disorders

Sleep disorders overlap with psychiatric problems – difficulty sleeping or excessive sleep are common symptoms and primary sleep disorders can worsen psychiatric problems. Disorders like narcolepsy, REM behaviour disorder and obstructive sleep apnoea respond to treatment. If there is significant decline in the person's functioning and a sleep disorder is suspected, an overnight sleep study can be diagnostic.

Assessment

History

A full account of psychiatric symptoms with special emphasis on the temporal sequence of events and their association with medical illness and treatment is warranted. Psychosocial history can offer clues that will help in tailoring a management plan and identifying precipitants.

Examination

Examination of the mental state is essential and the value of a thorough physical exam cannot be overstated. It helps to be aware of the symptoms and signs produced by damage to different regions of the brain (Table 6.2).

Table 6.2 Signs and symptoms resulting from damage to different parts of the brain.

Region of brain	Higher functions	Neurological localising signs
Frontal	Apathy and emotional lability, disinhibition, poor judgement	Primitive reflexes present, contralateral hemiplegia, Broca's aphasia (dominant hemisphere)
Temporal	Primarily memory	Wernicke's aphasia (dominant hemisphere)
Parietal	Calculation, perceptual and spatial orientation (non-dominant hemisphere)	Apraxia (dominant hemisphere), hemisensory disturbances, neglect. Gerstmann syndrome
Occipital	Perceptual and spatial orientation	Hemianopia

Investigation

Blood investigations, brain imaging and electrophysiology (electroencephalogram (EEG)) are all highly relevant.

Management

In the management of organic mental disorders, multidisciplinary and psychosocial treatments are as important as drug treatments. Close liaison with psychiatric and medical teams is required. Patients with neurological damage are more susceptible to side-effects of psychotropics, and also might be on a number of different medications that might interact, so caution is advised when prescribing. Medications like carbamazepine are enzyme inducers that can interfere with therapeutic levels of other medication. In the elderly, medication can be the cause for episodes of delirium.

When to refer to secondary care

Given the varied and unusual presentations of organic psychiatric disorders, patients tend to fall into grey areas between the medical and psychiatric services. A high index of suspicion is required when assessing patients with symptoms listed in Box 6.1, and early referral to secondary care for investigation and clarification of the diagnosis can reduce morbidity and improve quality of life in the longer term.

Key points

- Fluctuating consciousness, all hallucinations except auditory, and memory problems must raise suspicions of organic causes.
- Delirium is reversible, and associated with high mortality, so early recognition and treatment are essential.
- Dopaminergic and cholinergic medication (both agonists and blockers) can cause psychiatric side-effects.
- Psychosocial interventions including cognitive behavioural therapy, counselling and social support can make significant contributions to improving symptoms and preventing relapse.

■ People with organic mental health problems are more prone to side-effects from psychotropic medication and they should be monitored closely.

Further reading and bibliography

Kopelman, M. D. (2002) Disorders of memory. *Brain*, **125**, 2152–90.

Lishman, W. L. (1998) *Organic Psychiatry: the Psychological Consequences of Cerebral Disorder*, 3rd edn. Blackwell, Oxford.

Victor, M., Adams, R. D. and Collins, G. H. (1971). *The Wernicke–Korsakoff Syndrome*. F. A. Davis, Philadelphia.

World Health Organization (1992) *Tenth Revision of the International Classification of Diseases and Related Health Problems* (ICD-10). WHO, Geneva.

CHAPTER 7

Medically unexplained symptoms and chronic fatigue syndrome

Mohamed Abdelghani and Geoff Lawrence-Smith

Case history

A 42-year-old woman presented to her GP describing an eight month history of fatigue. During this period she visited her GP on numerous occasions with similar and related complaints. None of her blood tests showed any abnormalities that could explain her fatigue. For the past six months, she has taken sickness absence from her job as a laboratory researcher. The symptom of fatigue started after suffering from influenza shortly after being promoted at work. The promotion resulted in her being given responsibility for overseeing a major research project. She continued going to work for four days after developing flu but was encouraged by colleagues to visit her GP, who advised her to take two weeks' sick leave from work. As she did not want to delay the project she returned to work before fully recovering after staying at home for only one week. After returning to work she felt unable to stand for long hours in the laboratory, as she used to do, and started feeling increasingly fatigued with associated muscular pain. Her manager persuaded her to take further time off work. She spent most of this time at home sleeping and, when awake, tried to catch up with housework, but started feeling exceptionally fatigued on minimal physical exertion. The patient's husband was a journalist who spent a considerable amount of time abroad, leaving her to look after their two young children. Feeling unable to look after the children due to the fatigue led the patient to experience significant frustration and anxiety.

During the assessment the patient described feeling fatigued 'all the time'. She has to rest for almost a day after any physical or mental exertion. Resting does not make her feel better and, despite sleeping for up to ten hours each night and cat-napping during the day, she never feels refreshed. She complains of muscular pain throughout her body, persistent sore throat, difficulty concentrating and low mood.

After excluding potential medical causes for the patient's symptoms, the doctor diagnosed chronic fatigue syndrome (CFS) in light of her history and clinical presentation.

Introduction

Medically unexplained symptoms (MUS) are common in the general population and they are a frequent presentation to primary care. They include a number of disorders such as somatisation disorder (persistent and recurrent multiple physical symptoms), hypochondriacal disorder (preoccupation with one of more serious illnesses), chronic fatigue syndrome (physical and mental fatigue) and conversion disorders (loss of physical functioning). This chapter will mainly focus on chronic fatigue syndrome (also known as myalgic encephalitis), although the principles of management of these disorders is similar.

In secondary care, as many as two-thirds of patients attending general medical clinics do not receive an entirely biomedical explanation for their distressing symptoms. MUS appear more common in females and in younger age groups. Within the primary care setting, those suffering from MUS present in a variety of different ways. This can range from regular visits complaining of minor symptoms, to those with severe chronic fatigue syndrome, who may be bed-bound. Patients with MUS can provoke strong feelings among the health professionals who provide care for them. There is almost always a failure to explain the presenting symptoms according to any known pathology. Therefore patients may feel that they are not believed and that they are accused of making their symptoms up. Similarly, doctors can feel challenged due to their apparent lack of ability to explain the symptomatology (Hatcher, 2008).

While there is an inability to provide an explanation for MUS according to a wholly physical pathological process, it is widely accepted that symptoms arise due to the patient's misinterpretation of the significance of normal physical sensations, interpreting them instead as signs of disease. This concern leads to greater attention being paid to the sensations themselves, which in turn exaggerate the patient's concerns and anxieties. Such anxieties heighten the patient's sensation of somatic symptoms, thereby maintaining them in a vicious cycle. A typical example is the anxious or excited patient who becomes aware of their own heartbeat and subsequently worries that this signifies the development of heart disease. This can result in a change to the daily routine of activities, the request for medical investigations and the seeking of continuous reassurance that there is no cause for concern. In such cases, clear and effective communication by health professionals has an important role in countering the effects of such misinterpretations (Gelder, 2006).

Chronic fatigue syndrome (CFS) is a relatively common disease entity falling within the spectrum of MUS; a general practice with 10,000 patients is likely to have up to 40 patients with CFS. The physical symptoms of CFS can be as disabling as multiple sclerosis, systemic lupus erythematosus, rheumatoid arthritis and other chronic conditions (NICE, 2007).

Key aspects of history taking

As expected of all the psychiatric presentations, a comprehensive and detailed history should be taken. Such a detailed history is especially important in assessing MUS, and CFS in particular, in order to assess the numerous medical and psychiatric disorders which can present with symptoms overlapping with MUS/CFS. Due to the lack of diagnostic tests, a diagnosis of MUS/CFS is made by exclusion, thus underlining the indisputable importance of collecting a focused yet detailed history to exclude significant pathology. Such a history also provides the patient with an opportunity to explore their own symptoms with the doctor and often serves to validate their problems and cement a therapeutic and collaborative doctor–patient relationship.

Maintaining a patient-centred approach is essential in history-taking from a patient presenting with medically unexplained symptoms. This can be achieved in many different ways. A good start is to ensure that the symptoms are taken, initially at least, at face value, paying attention to how the symptoms affect the patient and his or her quality of life. Of particular importance is avoiding confrontation with the patient. Such confrontation is a risk, resulting in part at least, from frustration on the part of the doctor due to their inability to provide a biomedical explanation of the patient's symptoms.

In particular, when taking a history from a patient with suspected CFS, the doctor must be supremely confident of what symptoms to both elicit and exclude. Thus the importance of comprehensive knowledge of the appropriate diagnostic criteria cannot be overstated.

The most consistent features are fatigue that also occurs at rest and prolonged exhaustion, even after minimal physical or mental effort. At the same time other physical and cognitive symptoms, such as muscular pain and poor concentration, occur. Frustration and low mood also usually occur. People with CFS tend to avoid activity due to the fear of further fatigue.

Box 7.1 details the inclusion and exclusion criteria as they are listed in the NICE guidelines (2007).

In patients previously diagnosed with CFS, the diagnosis should be reconsidered if none of the following symptoms can be elicited:

- Post-exertion fatigue or malaise
- Cognitive problems
- Sleep problems
- Chronic pain

Box 7.1 NICE diagnostic criteria for chronic fatigue syndrome

Inclusion criteria
Clinically evaluated medically unexplained fatigue of **at least 6 months** that is:

- Of new onset (not life long)
- Not the result of ongoing exertion
- Not substantially alleviated by rest
- A substantial reduction in previous level of activities
- The occurrence of four or more of the following symptoms:
    - Subjective memory impairment
    - Sore throat
    - Tender lymph nodes
    - Muscle pain
    - Joint pain
    - Headache
    - Unrefreshing sleep
    - Post-exertional malaise lasting more than 24 hours

Exclusion criteria
- Active, unresolved or suspected disease
- Psychotic, melancholic or bipolar depression (but not uncomplicated major depression)
- Psychotic disorders
- Dementia
- Anorexia or bulimia nervosa
- Alcohol or other substance misuse
- Severe obesity

Mental state examination

Carrying out and documenting a mental state examination is fundamental for more than one reason. It should confidently permit the doctor to exclude the diagnosis of other mental disorders that might present with secondary fatigability, such as depression. The degree to which the patient holds unusual illness beliefs may reveal an underlying delusional disorder, treatable with antipsychotic medication. It is also vital to detect any secondary mental health difficulties that will need to be addressed during management. Insight should always be checked, as it will inform the management plan. The latter will depend on the patient's belief system, and what precisely the symptoms mean to the patient, so the doctor should explore the patient's acceptance of different modes of treatment and determine the extent to which the patient is capable of viewing the problem from a psychological perspective.

Physical examination

When patients present with MUS it is of huge importance that they receive an appropriate but comprehensive physical examination. It should be considered good practice to perform an examination at every appointment for the patient complaining of MUS. Such a physical examination serves three main functions:

- Relieves the patient's immediate anxiety that they have an acute medical problem
- Reinforces to the patient that their symptoms are being taken seriously
- Reassures the doctor that physical pathology has not been missed

When examining the patient with suspected or diagnosed CFS, the following clinical signs should prompt further investigation before attributing the symptoms entirely to the syndrome (NICE, 2007):

- Localising and focal neurological signs
- Signs of inflammatory arthritis or connective tissue disease
- Signs of cardiopulmonary disease
- Significant weight loss
- Sleep apnoea
- Clinically significant lymphadenopathy

Investigations

Although regular physical examination is useful, the potential for iatrogenic damage caused to people suffering from MUS due to over-investigation or both excessive and inappropriate treatment should never be underestimated. Over-investigation can be thought of as the 'dark side' of validating the patient's symptoms and runs the significant risk of increasing the 'illness behaviour' (Hatcher, 2008). However, a single standard set of bloods, including urea and electrolytes, full blood count, erythrocyte sedimentation rate and thyroid function tests, can once again reassure both doctor and patient.

Although there is no definitive investigation to diagnose CFS, initial investigations are useful within the diagnostic process. The function of such investigations is to enable the diagnosis to be made by exclusion (following negative results) of other causes as appropriate.

Box 7.2 outlines those investigations both recommended and discouraged by NICE (2007) in the diagnosis of CFS.

Management

The management of MUS is relatively universal, with minor alterations made to each treatment plan to take in to account the body system affected, the patient's particular concerns and any psychiatric comorbidity.

When constructing a management plan for the patient with MUS, the following should be considered.

Naming the problem

Once organic pathology has been excluded as far as possible it is very important to explain this to the patient and actively present the diagnosis of MUS or CFS to him or her. Whilst this may feel uncomfortable for the doctor, akin to an admission of failure to diagnose, the patient should be encouraged to accept the diagnosis in the knowledge that their physical health will continue to be monitored as new problems arise. The diagnosis should not be given in isolation but be an opportunity for psychoeducation, with appropriate time given for questions and signposting to resources. Through this form of empowerment the patient can learn more about the diagnosis and its implications for treatment etc. Useful resources include websites such as http://www.neurosymptoms.org/.

Box 7.2 Investigations for chronic fatigue syndrome

Tests to be done routinely

- Urinalysis for protein, blood and glucose
- Full blood count
- Urea and electrolytes
- Liver function
- Thyroid function
- Erythrocyte sedimentation rate or plasma viscosity
- C-reactive protein
- Random blood glucose
- Serum creatinine
- Screening blood tests for gluten sensitivity
- Serum calcium
- Creatine kinase
- Assessment of serum ferritin levels (children and young people only).

Tests *not* to be considered routinely

- The head-up tilt test
- Auditory brainstem responses
- Electrodermal conductivity

Tests *not* advised

- Tests for serum ferritin in adults, unless other tests suggest iron deficiency
- Test for Vitamin B12 deficiency or folate levels, unless a full blood count and mean cell volume show a macrocytosis
- Serological testing (unless there is a history indicative of infection)

Reframing the problem

It is necessary to attempt to shift the focus of the patient's concerns away from the isolated physical symptomatology towards accepting the significant role of psychological factors in physical illness and vice versa. While continuing to emphasise that the symptoms described are undoubtedly both real for the patient and familiar to the doctor, the focus of therapy may better be shifted towards coping with the symptoms using psychological techniques rather than waiting for the symptoms to resolve completely. Discussions surrounding general quality of life issues can be useful to encourage the patient to accept a more holistic package of care aimed at improving general wellbeing, thereby going some way to reducing the salience of the physical symptoms for the patient.

Psychological therapy

There are increasing provisions across the UK for psychological therapies, delivered through the Increasing Access to Psychological Therapies initiative. Cognitive behavioural therapy (CBT) has been shown to improve outcomes for patients with MUS. In anticipation of a referral for CBT, the patient should be encouraged to keep a diary of symptoms, corresponding mood states and associated stressors. This may help the patient to become more aware of how psychosocial factors impact on physical health. Activity scheduling can also be explored, again with the patient being encouraged to keep a diary of positive experiences and how they affect the physical symptoms. Such activity scheduling is especially useful for those with CFS, as well as graded exercise; although the latter should be planned whilst taking into account what outcome is truly realistic for the patient and explicitly including periods of rest. Simply advocating non-specific exercise or activity may simply set the patient up to fail and be detrimental for the patient with CFS.

Pharmacological therapy

Patients with comorbid psychiatric conditions should be considered for pharmacological therapy according to the relevant guidelines. Medications to manage pain would best be prescribed after advice from the local pain management clinic. The antidepressant duloxetine has been shown to reduce neuropathic pain, in addition to improving symptoms of depression, although further comparative data on effectiveness and cost analysis are needed.

Regular review

Finally, it is the experience of the authors that providing regularly scheduled appointments, with a doctor with whom the patient is familiar, even in the absence of new or recurring symptoms, appears to reduce the frequency of patients seeking advice and further investigations elsewhere (doctor-shopping).

It also improves the patient's sense of general wellbeing. Patients should be encouraged to use the planned appointments rather than repeatedly requesting urgent appointments with a duty doctor who may not be aware of the patient's condition. Whilst the prospect of such regular review may be daunting for an already busy GP, it must be borne in mind that, unlike malingering, the patient with MUS is not consciously fabricating symptoms for specific gain, but rather expressing their distress subconsciously through the body (somatisation). Understanding this concept is fundamental to the effective treatment of patients with MUS and CFS.

Key points

- Medically Unexplained Symptoms (MUS) are common in the general population and they are a frequent presentation to primary care.
- Patients with MUS can provoke strong feelings among the health professionals who provide care for them.
- Comprehensive and detailed history and physical examination provides the patient with an opportunity to explore their own symptoms with the doctor and often serves to validate their problems and cement a therapeutic and collaborative doctor–patient relationship.
- Over investigation can be thought of as the 'dark side' of validating the patient's symptoms and runs the significant risk of increasing the 'illness behaviour'.
- The management of MUS is relatively universal, with minor alterations made to each treatment plan to take in to account the body system affected, the patient's particular concerns and any psychiatric comorbidity.

Further reading and bibliography

Gelder, M., Harrison, P. and Cowen P. (2006) *Shorter Oxford Textbook of Psychiatry*, 5th edn. Oxford University Press, Oxford.

Hatcher, S. and Arroll, B. (2008) Assessment and management of medically unexplained symptoms. *British Medical Journal*, **336**, 1124–8.

Leader, D. and Corfield, D. (2007) *Why Do People Get Ill?* Hamish Hamilton, London.

NICE (2007) *Chronic Fatigue Syndrome/Myalgic Encephalomyelitis: Quick Reference Guide*. National Institute for Health and Clinical Excellence, London. http://guidance.nice.org.uk/CG53

Useful website

Functional and Dissociative Neurological Symptoms: a Patient's Guide: http://www.neurosymptoms.org/

CHAPTER 8

Mental health problems in women

Catherine Murgatroyd and Ruth Townsend

Case history

A 32-year-old married woman presents to the GP 16 weeks into her first pregnancy. She works as a successful business woman. She has a history of generalised anxiety disorder and two severe depressive episodes in 2002 and 2007, which responded to paroxetine. She recovered fully in between episodes and has remained on paroxetine. There is a strong family history of depressive disorder and anxiety.

On presentation to the GP she complains of feeling unable to cope with anything, not enjoying anything, feeling very low and tired, poor sleep with early morning waking and poor appetite. She also describes escalating anxiety about the pregnancy, feeling that she would not cope with a new baby and feeling desperately guilty about this. She has occasional suicidal thoughts, but had no desire to act on them, although these thoughts increased her level of guilt.

Introduction

This chapter outlines current thinking on the assessment and management of common mental illnesses during pregnancy, childbirth and in the postnatal period.

Women experience great emotional and physical changes during pregnancy and it is a time when mental health difficulties may emerge or worsen. It is increasingly recognised that mental health problems occurring during pregnancy and the postnatal period have a significant impact on the mother, and may also affect early bonding and the development of her child.

Women may not spontaneously disclose problems due to the cultural expectations placed upon them. It is therefore vital that active enquiries are made to anticipate and detect difficulties and that effective management strategies are in place. As pregnant women usually access the GP first, and the majority of common mental health problems emerging in the puerperium will be managed in primary care alone, such services clearly have an important role to play.

Epidemiology

Depression

The most common disorder is postnatal depression, occurring in about 13% of women; 3–5% have a moderately severe illness (Figure 8.1) and about 1.7% of these are referred to specialist mental health services. The majority of women with depression will be managed solely in primary care.

Similar numbers of women become depressed during pregnancy, as illustrated by the above case study. As approximately 50% of all people with depression are not identified, it is likely that depressed perinatal women are similarly unidentified and therefore not receiving optimum care.

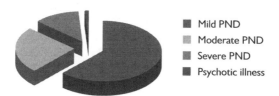

■ Mild PND
░ Moderate PND
■ Severe PND
■ Psychotic illness

Figure 8.1 The proportion of women with postnatal depression (PND) with varying severity.

Anxiety disorders

Anxiety disorders in pregnancy are probably almost as common as depression, but there is much less research. Such disorders would include post-traumatic stress disorder, obsessive compulsive disorder, generalised anxiety disorder and panic disorder. Around 15% of women have clinically significant levels of anxiety at 18 weeks pregnant. About half of these will continue to have such symptoms two months after giving birth.

Insomnia is common and although it is often due to pregnancy, rather than mental illness, it can exacerbate other mental health problems.

Psychotic illness

Rarer presentations, including puerperal psychosis (psychotic illness occurring within a month of birth), have an incidence of 1–2 women per 1000. The incidence is significantly increased in women with a personal history of bipolar affective disorder, a previous episode of puerperal psychosis or a family history. Women with pre-existing schizophrenia or schizoaffective disorder are also at risk of psychotic relapse after the birth.

Assessment and diagnosis

The approach to the assessment and diagnosis of common mental illness during pregnancy is the same as for mental illnesses occurring at any other time.

There has been much debate regarding screening for postnatal depression. The NICE guidelines (NICE, 2007) do not recommend the commonly used Patient Health Questionnaire (PHQ) or the Edinburgh Postnatal Depression Scale, and instead recommend the use of the Whooley questions (Whooley, 1997) (see Box 8.1). These questions should be routinely asked of all women on booking, regardless of their mental health history and could be used opportunistically by GPs or health visitors. Certain factors (see Box 8.2) have been shown to increase the risk of postnatal depression and these should also be asked about during the assessment.

An assessment of the degree of severity and risk, both of the current and past episodes, is essential as it dictates what management strategy to use and

Box 8.1 The Whooley questions

1. During the past month have you often been bothered by feeling down, depressed or hopeless?
2. During the past month have you often been bothered by having little interest or pleasure in doing things?
3. Would you like help with this?

Box 8.2 Risk factors for postnatal depression

- Depression and anxiety during pregnancy
- History of depression and anxiety
- Recent stressful life events
- Poor social support

whether a referral to secondary services is required. Referral should be considered for those with moderate to severe depression or anxiety, those with significant risk factors or those with untreated symptoms (see Box 8.3). Be warned that symptoms can escalate very quickly in the postnatal period and frequent reviews are recommended. Referral to children and families social services may also need to be considered if there is any concern about risk to children.

Box 8.3 'Red flags' – when to refer to secondary services

- Current mental state
- Suicidal ideation or self-harm
- Self-neglect
- Significant biological symptoms
- Escalating anxiety
- Rapidly worsening symptoms
- Thoughts of harming baby/unborn child
- Inability to cope with baby
- Negative thoughts – hopelessness, worthlessness, guilty thoughts
- Psychotic symptoms including unusual thoughts regarding baby
- Past history
- Significant mental illness, past episode of significant illness (e.g. BPAD, psychotic illness) especially in puerperium
- Suicide attempts and self-harm
- Social factors
- Lack of supportive partner/family
- Domestic abuse

Management

Psychological management

Even though there is good evidence for the efficacy of psychological treatments for common mental illness in general, there is scant research specifically into the efficacy and acceptability of psychological therapies for pregnant women. It is reasonable to assume that standard treatments would be just as effective for pregnant women, but standard services are not yet set up to deliver treatments in the prompt, flexible manner that would be required during this crucial time.

Prevention of postnatal depression

For pregnant women who have symptoms of depression and/or anxiety that do not meet diagnostic criteria, but do significantly interfere with personal and social functioning, NICE guidelines (2007) recommend that the health professionals should consider:

- If the woman has had a previous episode of depression or anxiety offer 4–6 sessions of cognitive behavioural therapy or interpersonal therapy.
- If no previous episode – increased level of social support (informal individual or group-based support).

For those who have no risk factors there is no benefit in offering treatment.

An encouraging development in the UK is the government-driven evaluation of the Family Nurse Partnership, an intensive multimodal nurse visiting programme for vulnerable families, originally developed in the USA. Trials have found significant short- and long-term benefits for families. There are currently 30 test sites running in the UK with more planned.

Psychological treatment for depression in postpartum period

More evidence (NICE, 2007) is available for treatment of depression in the postnatal period and the evidence base includes evaluation of CBT, interpersonal therapy (IPT) and psychodynamic psychotherapy, non-directive counselling (listening visits by health visitors) and social support (specific groups).

- All forms of treatment appear to be effective, with very little difference between them.
- Benefit is seen in both those with a diagnosis of depression and a high depression scale score, but treatment is more effective in those who have a formal diagnosis.
- There is some evidence that IPT may be more effective than psychoeducation (leaflets, audiotapes etc.), although this is not always the case.
- Six sessions of counselling appear to be more effective than just one.
- Psychoeducation with the partner is more effective than for the woman alone.
- Individual counselling is more effective than group counselling.

In terms of service provision and development, non-directive counselling is likely to be a cost-effective first line treatment option for women with mild to moderate depression in the postnatal period, compared with structured psychological therapy. The therapies are practically equal in terms of efficacy but there is a much higher discontinuation rate with structured work; women understandably find listening home visits more acceptable during the puerperium than visiting a clinic. Health visitors may therefore have an important role to play in performing listening visits for those with sub-threshold or mild to moderate symptoms.

Psychological treatments for those women with disorders other than depression

Home visiting for non-directive support may be beneficial for anxiety disorders and NICE recommends that the broad range of treatments identified in other NICE guidelines should be made available to women as appropriate.

Pharmacological management; prescribing for women of child bearing age

Medication is probably less acceptable, although no less effective, during pregnancy and lactation for women than at any other time. There are many aspects to take into consideration when prescribing antidepressants for a woman of childbearing age. It is essential to discuss the risks and benefits with the patient when considering commencing medication. The biggest concern for all is the risk that these medications may cause harm to the baby. When considering these risks, the available data are conflicting and can be difficult to access and understand. There are no randomised controlled trials involving pregnant woman and all psychotropic medications are prescribed off-licence in pregnancy.

Table 8.1 attempts to present a summary of the latest evidence in pregnancy and breast feeding for commonly used psychotrophic medications. It is important to remember that new research may change the recommendations and it may be necessary to check the latest evidence with the National Teratogenicity Service (http://www.toxbase.org/).

Principles of pharmacological management of common mental illness

The risks of pharmacological management must be weighed against the risks of not treating or stopping treatment. The risk of a severe depressive illness can be significant and relapse is common once an antidepressant is stopped. It is important to consider the consequences of deterioration, based on past psychiatric history and other risk factors. Severe depressive illness is associated with significant morbidity and mortality; suicide is currently the second leading cause of maternal death in the UK. The woman's ability to parent may be affected and her symptoms may affect all family members both directly and indirectly. A relapse may also affect her ability to engage in antenatal care, potentially leading to a poorer outcome.

In the majority of cases, the risk of leaving a severe depressive episode untreated because a woman is pregnant or breastfeeding is probably greater than any potential risk from an antidepressant. Thresholds for treating significant depression should not be any lower during pregnancy. Antidepressants are as effective for severe depression during pregnancy as at any other time and the majority of women will recover.

If pharmacological management is felt to be necessary and appropriate, a pragmatic approach is often required. Many women will present beyond the first trimester, meaning that the benefits of making a change in existing medication may be outweighed by the risk of relapse. Inadvertent exposure to any class of antidepressant is not an indication for invasive prenatal diagnosis techniques or termination, although an anomaly scan may be indicated following appropriate liaison with obstetric or neonatology services. General principles of prescribing apply; it is important to choose a medication that is likely to work, both in general for the condition and also to know what may have worked for this particular patient previously. It is equally important to know what did not work or caused unacceptable side-effects. A clear discussion with the patient must be documented and with other relevant professionals (e.g. midwife, obstetrician, neonatologist/paediatrician).

Table 8.1 Prescribing of psychotropic medication in pregnancy.

Drug	Properties
Tricyclic anti-depressants (TCA)	**Pregnancy** ■ Previously no reported teratogenicity based on large population studies (NICE, 2007) ■ Recent large study showed an association with TCA use in the first trimester and congenital malformations (Reis, 2010) ■ Amitriptyline and imipramine remain currently the most recommended (NICE, 2007) ■ No clear evidence to suggest an increased risk of miscarriage, equivocal data re: premature delivery and low birth weight **Breast feeding** ■ Secreted in breast milk, amitriptyline, nortriptyline clompipraime, dosulepin – low or unquantifiable levels ■ Generally few reports of adverse effects, those reported were transient **Neonatal complications** ■ Use in third trimester is associated with neonatal withdrawal symptoms (agitation, irritability, seizures, drowsiness, suckling problems); consider tapering and stopping ■ Less evidence for association with persistent pulmonary hypertension of the newborn than with SSRIs **General concerns** ■ Important side-effects include hypotension, constipation and sedation ■ Toxicity in overdose and potential risk to infant child if ingested
SSRIs	**Pregnancy** ■ Some association reported with premature birth, spontaneous abortion and low birth weight (NICE, 2007) ■ Increasing concern re: teratogenicity in first trimester. Several studies indicate a particular association with paroxetine and congenital heart defects with an increased risk from 1% (in the general population) to 2% (NICE, 2007). A recent study also found risk increased with sertraline and citalopram (Pedersen *et al.*, 2009) ■ Other studies have not found an increased risk with SSRIs in general or with paroxetine specifically ■ NICE guidelines (2007) advise avoiding paroxetine if possible ■ Fluoxetine is generally thought to be the safest of the SSRIs in terms of teratogenicity. Sertraline has the least placental exposure ■ Absolute risk remains very low for each individual mother **Breast feeding** ■ Fluoxetine and citalopram – higher levels excreted in breast milk than other SSRIs. No consistent evidence of adverse effects in exposed children ■ Sertraline and paroxetine – lowest levels found in breast milk compared with other antidepressants

Drug	Properties
	Neonatal complications ■ Neonatal withdrawal symptoms, usually mild and self-limiting ■ Increasing concern that SSRIs used after week 20 may be associated with an increased risk of the development of persistent pulmonary hypertension of newborn (risk increased from 1–2/1000 in general population to 6–12/1000 in those exposed (Chambers, 2006) ■ Aim to taper dose in third trimester, *but* risk of relapse **General concerns** Less toxic in overdose than TCAs
Monoamine oxidase inhibitors	■ Avoid due to maternal toxicity and lack of published data re safety
Others (e.g. venlafaxine, mirtazepine, duloxetine)	■ Should be avoided until more data available, withdraw cautiously and cross taper with safer alternative (NICE, 2007) ■ Higher rates of spontaneous abortion reported with venlafaxine, nefazodone and trazadone than SRRIs and TCAs (NICE, 2007) ■ Check latest advice before stopping/switching
Benzodiazepines	**Pregnancy** ■ Associations reported with increased risk of malformations if used in first trimester (e.g. cleft palate) but evidence is equivocal (NICE, 2007) ■ Third trimester use associated with floppy baby syndrome and withdrawal effects in neonates ■ Best advice is to avoid in pregnancy ■ In chronic use, pregnancy may be a good opportunity to withdraw if possible **Breast feeding** ■ May be excreted into breast milk but levels are low and concentration passed to infant probably insignificant
'Z drugs' – zopiclone/zolpidem	■ Little data on either pregnancy or breastfeeding ■ BNF advises to avoid ■ MHRA (2005) reported that infant may experience hypothermia and respiratory depression with zopiclone in third trimester
Antihistamines	■ Promethazine is widely used for insomnia but there is little data regarding its safety
Mood stabilisers	■ Sodium valproate, carbamazepine and lithium are associated with major congenital abnormalities and should be avoided if possible ■ Referral to specialist services will be required if these drugs are used or being considered
Antipsychotics	■ Typical antipsychotics (haloperidol and chlorpromazine) are the safest in pregnancy ■ Atypical antipsychotics are increasingly used in perinatal psychiatry services although there is little data on safety ■ Olanzapine is probably associated with increase in gestational diabetes ■ Very few data on depot antipsychotics and generally should be avoided but this will depend on risk of relapse

Other issues

Oral contraception

Consideration of contraception in the postnatal period is very important. An unplanned pregnancy may complicate any pre-existing mental health issues. If a woman is already struggling with mental health issues she may find one of the long-acting reversible contraceptives (LARCS) easier to manage than taking a pill every day or relying on condoms. Choice of contraceptive will be dictated in part by whether a woman is breast feeding, but most importantly by which method the woman feels will work for her. This may be influenced by her previous experience and the information she is given.

Women may have concerns that contraceptive medication may affect their mental health. All hormonal methods report low mood and loss of libido as side-effects. With the progesterone-only pill (POP), 'psychological disturbance, including depression' has been reported, but much less so than with the combined oral contraceptive pill (COCP). Depression and loss of libido are classed as relatively common side-effects of the COCP, but are generally minor and quickly reversible on stopping the medication. The IUD, as a non-hormonal method, does not have an effect on mood.

Child protection

Any clinician involved in the management of women during pregnancy and the post-partum period needs to have a thorough understanding of potential child protection issues. A risk assessment needs to be done not only for the new baby or child *in utero*, but also for any pre-existing children. Practitioners should ensure that they are familiar with the local child protection pathways and guidelines. Each Trust and social services department will have designated child protection leads and if there are any concerns regarding these issues appropriate referrals should be made. Communication between the different members of the multidisciplinary team involved in a woman's care is of paramount importance.

Organisation of perinatal mental health services

The structure of services is currently different in all areas of the country. Most services follow a 'stepped care model' (Table 8.2) with initial provision of brief low-intensity evidence-based treatments in primary care, followed by more intensive management as necessary. Perinatal psychiatry services are seeking to develop clear, integrated care pathways across all levels of the stepped care framework, with clear communication between all involved health professionals and continuity of care for patients.

Table 8.2 Stepped care model.

Tier	Health professionals	Roles
Primary care	GPs, primary care mental health workers, health visitors, primary care psychologists, counsellors	■ Detection of mental illness or significant risk factors ■ Management of mild to moderate mental illness, sub-diagnostic threshold symptoms, significant risk factors ■ Psychoeducation ■ Information about services ■ Liaison with secondary care services ■ 'Watch and wait' monitoring ■ Referral for primary care psychology/listening visits/social support ■ Consideration of pharmacological management ■ Consideration of safeguarding issues ■ Onward referral
Secondary care – maternity services	Midwives, obstetricians	■ Detection of mental illness or significant risk factors ■ Monitoring ■ Information sharing ■ Onward referral
Secondary care – general adult psychiatry	Psychiatrists, community psychiatric nurses, social workers, occupational therapists, psychologists	■ Management of moderate to severe symptoms, history of significant mental illness, treatment resistant illness, significant risk issues ■ Information sharing ■ Liaison ■ Consideration of safeguarding issues ■ Onward referral
Specialist perinatal psychiatry services – in development	To include: psychiatrists, community psychiatric nurses, psychologists, social workers	Specialist perinatal psychiatry services are being developed in response to growing concerns about meeting the needs of women during the perinatal period. These are not rolled out yet across the country and services often vary a great deal. Thresholds for referral vary. It is useful to check the referral criteria if services exist in the area. Most specialist services will be very happy to advise via telephone if necessary

Key points

- Mental health problems occur commonly in pregnancy and in the postnatal period.
- Primary care services have a key role in the detection and management of common mental illnesses.
- Management requires a complex risk benefit analysis and clear communication with all services involved.
- Specialist services are being developed; referral should be considered for those with moderate to severe illness.
- Safeguarding both the new born and other children in the household must never be forgotten.

References and further reading

Chambers, C., Hernandez Diaz, S., Van Marter, L. *et al.* (2006) Selective serotonin reuptake inhibitors and risk of persistent pulmonary hypertension of the new born. *New England Journal of Medicine*, **354**, 579–87.

NICE (2007) *Antenatal and Post Natal Mental Health*. Clinical guidelines 45. The National Instutute of Health and Clinical Excellence. http://guidance.nice.org.uk/.

Pedersen, L. H., Henricksen, T. B. *et al.* (2009) Selective serotonin reuptake inhibitors in pregnancy and congenital malformations: population based cohort study. *British Medical Journal*, **339**, b3569.

Reis, M. and Kallen, B. (2010) Delivery outcome after maternal use of antidepressant drugs in pregnancy; an update using Swedish data. *Psychological Medicine*, **5**, 1–11.

Whooley, M., Avins, A., Miranda, J. *et al.* (1997) Case finding instruments for depression. Two questions are as good as many. *Journal of General Internal Medicine*, **12**, 439–45.

Sexual disorders

Josephine Woolf and Margaret Denman

Case history 1

Melanie, a young-looking 25-year-old, looked nervous, making no eye contact with her GP. She had been referred by the practice nurse who had failed to take her smear test. After the usual form filling the doctor suggested that Melanie slip her lower things off and get on the couch. She did this slowly. Her knees were drawn up and she looked ashen and was shaking. By now the doctor was alerted to the fact that something was wrong and felt that she had to tread carefully. She therefore offered to do a one finger vaginal examination before proceeding with the speculum insertion. Melanie consented to this whilst turning her head to the wall. As the doctor moved her finger towards the vulva the patient flinched. Only the tip of the finger would go in. The doctor felt like an abuser and decided to stop. She commented that this seemed difficult and wondered if Melanie had difficulty with intercourse. She tearfully admitted that she had never had penetrative sex, despite being married for two years. She thought there was a 'blockage', as her husband could not get inside her.

After Melanie dressed, the doctor discussed the mechanism of vaginismus, explaining how she could explore for herself the relaxation and contraction of her muscles with her own finger. She arranged another appointment and assured her that the smear could be done in due course.

At the next appointment Melanie looked more grown-up and not quite so nervous. She had explored a bit with her finger and was happy for the doctor to try again. The doctor discussed Melanie's fantasy about her vagina and where this could have come from. She had not been sexually assaulted, but recalled an incident as a child when she fell on a bicycle and was taken to hospital because she was bleeding.

She reverted to a child as she discussed the humiliation and pain of the examinations. She felt damaged and exposed.

By looking together at this fantasy and gradually helping her overcome the vaginismus, Melanie was finally able to have penetrative intercourse. She came back a few months later to ask for her smear. The GP had concentrated on the feelings in the room, reflecting them back to the patient. She had not diverted into irrelevant and time-consuming history.

Case history 2

Angela and Jack came together to their GP. Although the appointment had been made in Jack's name, Angela took the chair next to the doctor and did all the talking whilst her husband looked sheepishly at the floor. They were in their early fifties and sex had been fine until recently – 'It's all Jack's fault', she said emphatically. 'He can't keep an erection – I want you to examine him and find out what's wrong'. She crossed her arms and looked at the doctor expectantly. The doctor, who knew them both well, felt hopeless and inadequate. Realising that he felt impotent before this powerful and demanding woman, he asked her to go to the waiting room while he examined her husband. She agreed reluctantly.

Once she had gone Jack started to talk. 'You know what she's like', he said. Without colluding the GP asked him to explain. She bosses me around all the time. It is worse now the kids have left home. I never get a moment to myself. She is always asking me to do something. The doctor pointed out what was happening and that his penis was rebelling even if he couldn't do so in any other way. They established that there was no physical problem, as masturbation was fine. A genital examination was also reassuring.

After talking to his doctor, Jack had the courage to discuss things with Angela and to stand up to her. Gradually his erection improved and they resumed intercourse. The doctor had used the impotent feelings that he had experienced when Angela was in the room and reflected this back to Jack. Coupled with the reassurance that this was not a physical problem, the patient was able to work the rest out.

Introduction

Sexual problems are difficult to talk about. Patients will often 'test out' their doctor before disclosing a problem which they may see as embarrassing or shameful. Box 9.1 lists sexual problems that may be encountered by GPs.

Box 9.1 Sexual problems presenting in general practice

Common problems

Men	Women
Erectile dysfunction (ED)	Vaginismus/non-consummation
Loss of libido	Loss of libido
Premature ejaculation (PE)	Dyspareunia
Delayed/non-ejaculation	Anorgasmia
Testicular/prostatic pain	'Can't feel anything'

Less common problems (men and women)

Sexual aversion

Paraphilias: fetishism, sado-masochism, paedophilia, exhibitionism

Sexual addiction; pornography addiction

Gender dysmorphia

Body dysmorphophobias, e.g. penis size, labial size

GPs should be able to pick up subtle or covert messages. They must be open-minded and receptive to sexual difficulties and should encourage and facilitate discussion without embarrassment. The 'hand on the door' at the end of a consultation for something else (easy escape) could be managed with a firm follow-up date and an assurance that this is an important problem which justifies its own appointment.

Assessment

History

The history should be patient-centred, not doctor-centred: allow the patient to tell the story as they wish. Observe body language: appearance, eye contact and attitude. Note evidence of feelings: anxiety, anger, depression, sadness, irritation. Look for defences: rudeness, jokeyness, 'I don't care', over-familiarity; they may compensate for feelings of vulnerability, inadequacy or exposure. Almost anything is easier to talk about than a sexual problem!

If you can comment – 'You seem worried/angry/sad' – this may free the patient to tell you more. Similar reflections, observations and open-ended questions will give you more information than closed questions. Silence can be effective, giving the patient space to tell their story.

Presentation may be overt or covert. Covert presentations include: recurrent vaginal discharge with negative swabs ('I need you to look at me down there, something feels wrong'); failure to attend for smears or inability to allow the smear to be taken ('I am afraid of pain – I have a block'); failure to find any suitable contraceptive method ('Sex isn't good – I can't face talking about it').

It is helpful to know: why has the patient come now for help? Is this a primary or a secondary problem? If secondary, what was sex like before? Was there an obvious triggering event: a change of partner, surgery, a baby, an assault, a death, an illness, moving in together? Box 9.2 lists transition points when sexual problems may occur. What is the relationship like with the partner? What is the usual frequency of intercourse? How long is it since the last intercourse? What about masturbation? Orgasm? Fantasies? – asking about these is often surprisingly helpful.

For men with erectile dysfunction or premature ejaculation, what was the usual length of time to ejaculation before the problem began? Does it occur with a partner but not with masturbation (situational)? Are morning erections fine or is the erectile dysfunction global (occurring in all situations)? Was the onset slow, over months or years (more likely to be physical) or rapid – days, even overnight (much more typical of a psychological cause)?

Clues in the history may point towards physical causes. In particular, erectile dysfunction may be associated with cardiovascular disease; diabetes is a well-known cause. Enquire about medicines, alcohol consumption, smoking and recreational drugs. Is the patient depressed (associated with loss of libido)? Don't forget to ask men on beta blockers or other drugs such as antidepressants if they are experiencing sexual problems; they may be reluctant to complain.

Be aware of changes in the atmosphere during the consultation, maybe a hint of tears, a loss of eye contact, a lightening or darkening of mood, an increase or release of tension. What was being discussed at the time? What does this reveal?

Examination

Physical examination is important because it may reveal feelings, fantasies and fears as well as the presence or absence of pathology. You need to understand the underlying anxiety; reassurance without this understanding is ineffective, even if you think the genitals are normal.

Box 9.2 Potential problem times when sexual difficulties may appear or be unmasked

Teens and twenties
Lack of self-confidence, not 'ready' for sex, possible child sexual abuse, searching for love through sex, poor parental role modelling (especially mothers), bad first sexual experience.

Marriage
Boredom after lust has waned, lack of privacy if others in the house (e.g. in-laws), failure of relationship, lack of communication, inability to express needs. Financial difficulties. Betrayal, loss of trust.

Planning pregnancy
Non-consummation or non-ejaculation revealed. Infertility investigations and treatment causes sexual tension. Guilt and sadness following termination of pregnancy (TOP) or miscarriage.

Childbirth
Sense of failure if medical intervention needed. Feelings of exposure and loss of dignity at delivery. Tiredness, loss of sexiness, total involvement with baby. No time for self, no time for couple, no fun. Perceived conflict between being a good mother and a lover. Men: trauma having witnessed birth. Feelings of exclusion, anger.

Loss of fertility
Disease, surgery, cancer. Menopause.

Mid-life
Children's adolescence, elderly parents' dependency. Menopause with its physical and emotional manifestations. Gynaecological surgery. Divorce. Redundancy. Feeling 'past it'. Regrets, sadness of what has been missed. New relationships, different sexual needs.

Examination must be sensitive; give the patient privacy to undress, ensure they are comfortable on the couch, provide something to cover them up and ensure there is a screen. Consider a chaperone, but be aware that a disclosure may not occur with a third person present.

If there is refusal or avoidance of examination, or repeated non-attendance for smears: explore the reason for this. Is it fear? Shame? Explore why she (he) is reluctant, rather than insisting it be done now.

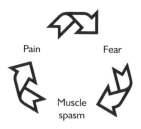

Pain   Fear

Muscle
spasm

Figure 9.1 The vicious cycle of vaginismus.

Observe body language, facial expression and attitude during the examination. Beware of taking comments at face value. A woman having a smear might remark, 'What a horrible job you have, doc!', revealing her own feelings of disgust about her body. Better to say, 'It sounds as though you don't really like that part of you', than, 'No I love my job!'.

If there is evidence of fear, try to uncover what it is before looking and touching. What is the fantasy about what is wrong, or what happened at childbirth or operation or during an assault? Behaviour and feelings revealed on the couch reflect behaviour with the partner, e.g. detachment, terror, anger, defensiveness, passivity, submissiveness or control. Vaginismus may arise because of fear of pain, as a reflex protective mechanism (see Figure 9.1). However, it may also be a somatic response to the (unconscious) desire to shut the partner out, an angry gesture.

Be aware of the vulnerability of the patient during examination; clothes are off, defences are down. This may lead to disclosure – the 'moment of truth'. Allow a moment to let tears fall, to hold and contain the distress and pain, – but plan an 'exit strategy' – perhaps acknowledge the importance of what has been revealed and make definite follow-up arrangements.

Examining women

Vulval inspection – a mirror for the patient to see for herself may be useful if she is uncertain about her anatomy.

Use a gentle one-finger examination at her pace to let her feel in control. Use two fingers if it is not painful. If she has vaginismus, explain how she can relax her vaginal muscles (levators) by pretending to stop and start peeing, which brings these involuntary muscles under conscious control (Kegel exercise) (Hay-Smith and Dumoulin, 2006). Encourage self-examination to confirm normality, and be in touch with a part of her body she does not know, is afraid of or has been ignoring.

Examining men

As with women, this is important as it may enable them to reveal their deepest secrets. Feelings about the genitals may emerge when they are not wrapped up in clothes and defences.

If he lies on the couch, you will be above him; if he stands and you sit to examine him, he is above you. Which would be better for him? For you? You might choose the first option if you find him a bit threatening; the second option may be better for a man with poor self-esteem and a dominant partner who makes him feel small.

A man embarrassed to show his genitals to a doctor may reflect his anxiety or shame with a partner.

Occasionally a man may sexualise a consultation – flirting or getting an erection during the examination. There are a number of possible reasons for this, one of which is to deprofessionalise the doctor to avoid looking at the real sexual problem he has. He can make himself feel more potent by diminishing the doctor's authority and control. A skilled doctor can see through this and must assert his or her professional status (whilst perhaps even giving him credit for his normally functioning organ!) in order to help him identify the problem. (See note on IPM training, below.)

Investigations

Baseline tests to exclude diabetes, thyroid deficiency and alcohol excess should be done as indicated. Remember that erectile dysfunction may be a symptom of cardiovascular disease.

Testosterone is rarely below normal in younger men (under 40). Testosterone should be measured at around 9:00 a.m. when levels are at their highest. Sex hormone binding globulin (SHBG) should be measured to give an indication of free (active) testosterone. If low, consider measurement of follicle stimulating hormone (FSH), luteinising hormone (LH) and prolactin to distinguish primary testicular failure (FSH high, testosterone low) from possible pituitary tumour (FSH and LH low, testosterone low, prolactin possibly high).

Management

Listening, allowing the patient to 'unload' and to understand and get things in perspective is a major part of therapy. Patients can often work the rest out for themselves. Don't worry about 'opening a can of worms' – a few minutes will suffice and you can arrange early follow-up.

Sexual problems are never 'all in the mind'; the mind and body are inextricably linked, and both should be attended to.

Hormone treatment is rarely needed, but sometimes testosterone helps in men with low levels. Menopausal women may respond to hormone replacement therapy and vaginal oestrogens may help with vaginal discomfort. There is limited evidence for the use of testosterone in women and it is currently licensed only for women post-oophorectomy also on oestrogen.

Patients sometimes need help in learning to communicate their needs to their partner. Remind them of the need to set aside special time for each other, to keep sexual times fun and stimulating; 'practising' should not feel like a chore.

Sometimes it is better to make definite follow-up arrangements than offer an open invitation to return; patients may feel their problem is too trivial to waste your time; they need to know that you feel it is worthwhile making another appointment. Two or three ten minute slots can achieve as much as an hour of 'specialist' time.

Behavioural therapy

There is a role for basic behavioural therapy. Vaginismic women can examine themselves with a finger, practise relaxing their levator muscles (see 'Examining women' above), slowly increasing to two fingers, then their partner's fingers, and then progressing to full penetration.

Some women find graded vaginal trainers helpful. If a woman cannot manage with fingers this is a good alternative. The disadvantage is that it is more difficult to know exactly how effective she is in trying to relax her muscles. It may also feel too 'mechanical'. Why not use a vibrator instead, which is more fun? Amielle Comfort vaginal trainer sets (Owen Mumford) are available on prescription and online.

For men with premature ejaculation, stop-start, withdrawal and squeeze techniques can be of help in learning to control and delay the time to ejaculation. Starting with masturbation, when they will be less anxious, they can then ask their partner to help, initially manually, then during full penetrative intercourse.

Masters and Johnson's (1970) behavioural techniques have been widely used, particularly in the context of performance anxiety. They consist of graded touching exercises, beginning with non-erotic areas (and forbidding sexual touch at this stage) and slowly progressing to massage and caressing of erogenous zones. However, these require regular follow-up arrangements and may be better left to a different agency, such as Relate (see below).

Treatment for physical problems in men

If the cause of erectile dysfunction is thought to be physical there are a variety of treatments available. Sometimes drug treatment is also used when there is a psychological or mixed problem as it can help return confidence. Regulations regarding availability on the NHS and the dosages of preparations are clearly laid out in the British National Formulary.

The most commonly used drugs are the phosphodiesterase type-5 inhibitors, the best known being sildenafil (Viagra). They cannot be used in men also taking nitrates and in those who are at very high risk of a cardiac event. In general men able to climb two flights of stairs at a reasonable rate without angina are fit enough for moderate sexual activity. Vardenafil is shorter acting and may be useful if there is a risk of side-effects such as flushing or headache. Tadalafil is much longer-acting, having some effect for up to 24 hours. Its absorption is affected less by food and can allow more spontaneity and more opportunity on a cost-restricted prescribing regime. Tadalafil at a lower dose can be used daily. Men with diabetes are resistant to these drugs and often need the highest doses. It is worth trying different preparations and persisting. Men with neurological disorders are far more sensitive to these drugs and lower doses should be used initially.

If these drugs fail then intraurethral or intracavernosal alprostadil can be tried. The latter may need specialist intervention as men need to be shown how to inject into the penis. Diabetics on insulin may be more adept at this than others. Side-effects are common and there needs to be provision for treatment of priapism that occurs rarely. There is some evidence that drugs such as paroxetine, sertraline, clomipramine and to a lesser extent fluoxetine can help with premature ejaculation (Waldinger, 2004). Delayed ejaculation is of course a side-effect of these drugs.

The vacuum pump is very useful and should not be forgotten. It can be prescribed free of charge for diabetics and others meeting the criteria for NHS prescription. Some men who get erections that are not maintained can manage with a penile ring. These mechanical devices can be obtained via the internet, mail order or on prescription.

Brief psychodynamic therapy

This approach has been developed by the Institute of Psychosexual Medicine (IPM) for primary care doctors to use in the short time slot available to them. Brief psychodynamic and interpretive skills involve active listening and an understanding of the patient's problem via an awareness of the relationship between the doctor and the patient in the consulting room.

Genital symptoms as presented to the doctor may be expressions of under-lying – and often unconscious – feelings, e.g. shutting out the partner (vaginis-mus), shutting off from painful feelings ('I can't feel anything'), helplessness (erectile impotence) or anger (erectile impotence – 'downing tools and going on strike') or anorgasmia (inability to let go).

Behaviour in the consulting room with the doctor reflects behaviour at home with the partner. Unconscious feelings may come to light through trans-ference phenomena, where the doctor is made to feel what the patient is feel-ing, for example helpless, impotent, angry, bored. Helping patients understand, acknowledge and verbalise these feelings enables them to begin a process of change with their partner. Feelings can be openly discussed, instead of being expressed as a sexual problem.

The genital examination is also a psychosomatic event, and an ideal time to explore feelings. Defences are lowered and pain may be revealed as being emotional in origin, even if physical in manifestation. Fears and fantasies about the body may be revealed. The doctor's feelings during the examination (for example like an abuser) provide valuable clues to the patient's feelings (as someone who has been abused?) and a reflection of this insight to the patient may facilitate disclosure. The genital examination, sensitively done, is often the most important part of the therapy.

Every individual is unique, with a unique set of problems. The doctor is not the expert, but starts each new encounter in ignorance with the patient, and they work together to understand the problem. The patient takes responsibility, rather than expecting the doctor to provide all the answers.

The IPM offers training courses for doctors through Balint-style seminars. Information is available on the website: http://www.ipm.org.uk/.

When to refer

It is often hard for a GP to decide when to refer a patient with a sexual prob-lem. This will depend to some extent on the services available in their area and their own skills. Loss of libido and other sexual problems can often be due to a relationship difficulty and referral to Relate may be appropriate. Relate also have sex therapists who work in a behavioural way, suiting some highly motivated couples. If a patient has mental health problems they may need to be referred to the community mental health team or to the practice counsellor, depending on the severity. The counsellor may also be able to deal with other issues that may be affecting a person's sex life. Sometimes more specific types of counselling are required, e.g. after rape or childhood sexual abuse. Doctors trained by the IPM are available in many areas to take referrals.

Physical problems in men and women can be dealt with by many GPs, especially with intra- practice referral. Sometimes female patients may need to see a gynaecologist or vulval specialist. A male patient not responding to simple treatments may need referral to a urologist or specialist erectile dysfunction clinic, either for investigation or initiation of alprostadil injections.

Referral to psychologists for cognitive behavioural therapy for paraphilias may be appropriate. There are specialist clinics for transgender patients.

Key points

- Patients will disclose their sexual problems if they sense you are willing and interested to hear them.
- Do not be afraid to ask about sex.
- Attend to the body and the mind – they are always linked.
- Unless the real reason for anxiety about a sexual problem is known reassurance will be futile.
- Significant therapeutic interventions can occur within a short time.

Further reading and bibliography

Hay-Smith, E. J., Dumoulin, C. (2006) Pelvic floor muscle training versus no treatment, or inactive control treatments, for urinary incontinence in women. *Cochrane Database of Systematic Reviews (Online)* (1): CD005654. doi: 10.1002/14651858.

Masters, W. H. and Johnson, V. E. (1970) *Human Sexual Inadequacy*. Bantam Books, Toronto, New York.

Waldinger, M. D. *et al.* (2004) Relevance of methodological design for the interpretation of efficacy of drug treatment for premature ejaculation: systematic review and meta-analysis. *International Journal of Impotence Research*, **16**, 369–81.

Skrine, R. and Montford, H. (eds.) (2001) *Psychosexual Medicine, an Introduction*. Arnold, London.

Useful website

Relate: http://www.relate.org.uk/

CHAPTER 10

Mental health problems in children

Helen Bruce and Benjamin Keene

Case history 1

Alex is a 7-year-old boy whom his mother has brought to the surgery as she is having difficulty managing his behaviour. Alex is constantly 'on the go'. He fidgets all the time and will not sit still. Alex does not seem to listen when you are talking to him, he cannot wait his turn, and when his mother takes him shopping he will run around causing chaos, making it almost impossible to get the shopping done. He is impulsive and will dart across roads with no warning. Alex is very different from his brother, who is just a year younger than him but already seems more responsible. His mother feels exhausted trying to manage him.

Alex's teachers have always said that he is a 'live wire' since nursery and he is often in trouble for his behaviour and not sitting still. The teachers are now concerned that his poor concentration and inability to sit still are affecting his school work.

Introduction

Child mental health problems are common but respond well to early intervention and treatment, making it important that they are recognised and managed appropriately in general practice, with onward referral to specialist services when required. Recognition itself is challenging, especially in the adolescent age group who may be reluctant to disclose mental health worries. Any young person who has co-existing medical problems, neurological problems, a neurodevelopmental condition, learning difficulties or who is a looked-after child (cared for by the local authority, e.g. in a foster placement) is at a greater risk of child mental health problems and should warrant careful assessment.

This chapter considers the assessment of child psychiatric disorders, common disorders that may be seen in general practice, when to refer to secondary services or other agencies and some general principles for management. Two of the most common conditions that GPs are likely to see, Attention Deficit Hyperactivity Disorder (ADHD) and depression, are then considered in more detail and other key conditions briefly. Key learning points are listed at the end of the chapter.

Assessment of child and adolescent psychiatric disorders

When assessing a child or adolescent, it is usually helpful to meet with the whole family at the start of the interview, but at some stage in the assessment, both the parent(s) and the young person should be seen individually if this is at all possible in the general practice situation.

The family interview should begin by putting the family at their ease. What do the family see as the problem and how is it affecting their lives? How are they trying to deal with it at present? What help have they already received?

With the younger child, it may not be formally possible to assess the child's mental state and the clinician will need to rely on their observations. Key things to consider are shown in Box 10.1.

It is important to obtain from the parent(s) a thorough description of the current problem and an account of the child's development, medical and school history. The key information from the history is summarised in Box 10.2.

At the end of the interview with the child, a helpful technique is to ask the child 'if you had three wishes what would you wish for?'. The child will often give useful information about their situation, fears and worries, using terms that are meaningful to them.

With an adolescent, it is important to pay attention to risk assessment and to respect their individual autonomy and confidentiality. They may have a very different view of a presenting problem or risk issue to that of their family. A psychiatric mental state examination should be carried out as in Box 10.1 and it is usually possible to focus more on symptoms than with a younger child. Symptoms of psychosis should also be excluded as well as gaining some understanding of the young person's insight into their difficulties.

Box 10.1 Observing the child (adapted with permission from Bruce and Evans (2008))

- Behaviour
  - Appearance
  - Emotional state
  - Mannerisms and gestures
  - Any hyperactivity
- Talk
  - Form
  - Content
- Anxiety and mood
  - Fears and worries
  - Disturbed or aggressive
  - Withdrawn or shy
  - Sadness
- Interactions
  - Parent–child
  - Interaction with other family members
  - Interaction with interviewer
- Intellectual function
  - Level of ability-consistent with chronological age?

Box 10.2 Information from the parent(s) – (adapted with permission from Bruce and Evans (2008))

- What is the problem and how does it affect the child/family
- Behavioural problems
- Emotional symptoms
- Attention and concentration
- Any hyperactivity
- School history, academic achievement, attendance, peer relationships
- Family life and relationships
- Family history of illness
- Any recent trauma
- Developmental history
- Medical history
- The child's strengths
- What help/interventions have already been tried
- What interventions have been successful

Physical examination and investigations

Most children presenting with psychological difficulties in general practice should also routinely have a physical examination. Reasons for this include the possibility of an underlying undetected physical condition or the prescription of medication that could have physical side-effects.

Other sources of information

Even when assessing a child in a busy GP practice it is important to try to obtain, with parental consent, information from other agencies involved with the child and especially the school.

Formulation

First of all, the clinician will need to consider whether the child's behaviour, emotional state or presenting difficulty is abnormal. Is a symptom abnormal in relation to a child's age and gender, culture, developmental stage, severity and frequency? Is the symptom leading to functional impairment in the everyday life of the child?

A formulation of the child's difficulties will require the clinician to piece together the presenting features of the problem, with any aetiological factors, and to comment on the differential diagnosis, management and prognosis. This evaluation will form the basis on which any intervention is planned.

Common disorders of childhood and adolescence

The most common disorders seen in children and adolescents are listed in Box 10.3.

General principles in the management of child psychiatric disorders

It is important to discuss the condition, its symptoms and their management with the young person, their family and the school, with permission, as this

Box 10.3 Common disorders in childhood and adolescence

Childhood
- ADHD
- Autistic spectrum disorders
- Obsessive compulsive disorders
- Tics and Tourette's syndrome
- Fears and phobias
- Specific learning disabilities
- Specific language impairments
- Disorders of attachment
- School attendance difficulties
- Suspected abuse
- Emotional disorders

Adolescence
- Deliberate self-harm
- Anxiety disorders
- Obsessive compulsive disorders
- Post-traumatic stress disorders
- Substance misuse
- Psychotic illness
- Eating disorders
- Emerging personality disorders
- Depression

usually results in a reduction of anxiety and improvement in the symptoms. Supporting the parents and/or school in the implementation of simple behavioural management, e.g. positive reinforcement of desirable behaviour, is essential. Always liaise with other agencies involved with the child, with the family's consent, so that a consistent approach can be taken in any behavioural management strategies. Ongoing risk assessment and parental support must be a key part of every review.

When to refer to secondary services

Box 10.4 and Table 10.1 below show when to refer to secondary services and when to refer to other agencies.

Case example

Alex is showing the triad of symptoms of Attention Deficit Hyperactivity Disorder (ADHD) of hyperactivity, impulsivity and poor concentration. His mother is exhausted and his school work is suffering. You decide to refer to secondary services for an ADHD assessment.

Box 10.4 When to refer to secondary services

- When a child is causing undue concern
- When primary care options are not working
- Suicidal intent (early referral)
- Psychotic features or suspicion of early onset psychosis (early referral)
- Eating disorders (early referral)
- School refusal (early referral)
- Severe behavioural problems
- Moderate to severe depression, anxiety or obsessive compulsive disorder
- Moderate to severe post-traumatic stress disorder
- Moderate to severe phobias, tics and Tourette's
- Assessment of ADHD and other neurodevelopmental disorders (depending on local protocols)
- Assessment of autistic spectrum disorders (depending on local protocols)

Table 10.1 When to refer to other agencies.

Condition/issue	Agency
Suspected abuse	Child protection services
Risk of harm to others	Consider police
Substance misuse	Substance misuse services
Specific learning difficulties, e.g. dyslexia	Educational psychology
Coordination problems	Occupational therapy
Employment issues/career issues	Connexions

Attention Deficit Hyperactivity Disorder (ADHD)

ADHD is a condition characterised by symptoms in three key areas:

- **Hyperactivity**
  Children may leave their seat or fidget constantly when they are supposed to be completing a task. They appear to have more 'energy' than others, but cannot channel this into their work or play.
- **Impulsivity**
  These children cannot tolerate waiting for what they need and will push into a queue or not understand the concept of raising a hand to answer a question. Conflicts with other children may frequently get out of control and become violent.
- **Inattention**
  These children are often distracted from their task and can often only manage up to ten minutes before losing focus. They cannot watch through the whole of a television programme or video or play a computer game for a long period of time, even if it is an activity that they enjoy.

ADHD is a dimensional, not a categorical, disorder and diagnosis is made at a point where there is impairment (psychological, social and functional) in multiple settings – most often at school and at home. Many criticisms of ADHD focus on the fact that these behaviours are sometimes exhibited by children that do not have ADHD. We all expect seven-year-old children to run around – it is the qualitative difference in behaviour that is crucial in making the diagnosis.

ADHD usually affects boys. The sex ratio is approximately 3:1, with prevalence rates of 1–3%.

Initial concerns are often raised by the child's school who will refer on to CAMHS/primary care for further assessment. At this early stage, parents should be offered education and training on modifying behaviour informed by social learning theory.

The formal diagnosis and treatment of ADHD should be left to specialist services using detailed histories, rating scales and school observations. See Table 10.2 for management strategies recommended by NICE (2008).

Although medication is initiated by specialist services, continued prescribing and monitoring can be carried out in primary care. Given concerns about stunted growth with psychostimulants (e.g. methylphenidate), NICE (2008) recommend that height and weight be monitored every 6 months. Heart rate and blood pressure should be monitored every 3 months and before and after dose changes. Doctors should be aware of potential adverse effects affecting sexual dysfunction, seizures, abnormal movements and psychotic symptoms.

Table 10.2 NICE (2008) recommendations for management of ADHD.

Service	Mild impairment	Moderate impairment	Severe impairment
Primary care	Watchful waiting Parent training/education initiatives Referral to specialist services if impairment persists		Parent training/education initiatives Referral to specialist services for formal assessment and diagnosis
Specialist care	Assessment and diagnosis	Assessment and diagnosis Group or individual psychological therapy	Assessment and diagnosis Pharmacological management (methylphenidate recommended initially)

Referrals to specialist services for ADHD

- Assessment and diagnosis
- Those with moderate/severe impairment of functioning

Depression

Depression in young people is heterogeneous and is often comorbid with other mental health difficulties – anxiety disorders, conduct disorder and ADHD. The prevalence of depression in primary school age children is estimated to be 1–2%, rising to 3–8% in adolescents. Before the onset of puberty, depression is more common in boys, but the opposite is the case after puberty and into adult life.

The symptoms in children mirror those in adults – lack of interest in normal activities, persistent low mood, altered sleep and lack of appetite. These often manifest as boredom in school, getting in trouble for not paying attention and more frequent disputes with siblings and parents. Other specific risk factors include a history of bullying or parental depression, and family-related factors (e.g. marital discord and separation).

Table 10.3 summarises the guidance on the management of depression in children and young people from NICE (2005). There is evidence that SSRI antidepressants can increase the intensity of suicidal feelings in young people and NICE (2005) recommends caution in their use, preferring psychological therapies. Young people should also be discouraged

Table 10.3 Summary of NICE (2005) recommendations on the management of depression in children.

Management	Mild depression	Moderate/severe depression
First line	Watchful waiting: no active treatment but regular assessment	Specialist assessment by CAMHS professional Psychological intervention
Second line	Non-directed supportive therapy, group CBT, guided self-help	Alternative/additional psychological therapy Augment psychological therapy with fluoxetine (maximum dose 20 mg)

from taking St John's Wort, as this has an unknown side-effect profile, no evidence supporting its use and is known to interact with other medications, including contraceptives.

Since the publication of NICE guidance (2005), there has been further research into the treatment of moderate/severe depression in young people. This has suggested that the best response is achieved when combination therapy is used, i.e. CBT together with fluoxetine.

When to manage in primary care

- Mild depression without comorbidity
- Recent undesirable life events without history of depression or ideas of self-harm

When to refer to specialist care

- Moderate or severe depression
- Active ideas of suicide
- Depression in the context of established familial history of depression
- Mild depression that has not responded to primary care interventions

Other childhood disorders

Autism

Autistic spectrum disorders classically have a triad of abnormal social development, communication and restricted interests. Language development is delayed, although this does not feature in Asperger's Syndrome. Management is based upon optimising educational and social support to the child and family and using behavioural therapy to reduce any abnormal behaviours.

Separation anxiety

This is a disorder specific to childhood and is a fear of separation from the primary care-giver due to the belief that something devastating will happen to them. This, along with other anxiety disorders (many of which present similarly to adult anxiety disorders), is best treated with behavioural or psychological therapy.

School refusal

School refusal is another anxiety disorder which often presents at times of school transition (aged 5 or 11) with refusal to attend school. This too may be related to separation anxiety, may represent a school phobia or be a result of bullying or a fear of academic failure. It is managed by an early return to school along with close communication with teachers.

Key points

- Child mental health problems are common and respond well to early intervention and treatment.
- Consider whether the child's behaviour, emotional state or presenting difficulty is abnormal in relation to a child's age and gender, culture, developmental stage. Is the difficulty persistent, severe and frequent enough to be considered abnormal?

- Consider whether the symptom is leading to functional impairment in the everyday life of the child. Is it interfering with the child's development, causing social restriction, distress to the child or others?
- Information must be gathered from the child, family and other sources, e.g. school.
- If you suspect abuse, contact children's social services.

Further reading and bibliography

Bruce, H. and Evans, N. (2008) Assessment of child psychiatric disorders. *Psychiatry: Child Psychiatry*, **7**, 242–5.

Harrington, R. (2005) Assessment of psychiatric disorders in children. *Psychiatry*, **4**, 19–22.

NICE (2005) *Depression in Children and Young People: Identification and Management in Primary, Community and Secondary Care.* Clinical guidelines CG28. National Institute for Clinical and Health Excellence, London. http://guidance. nice.org.uk/CG28.

NICE (2008) *Attention Deficit Hyperactivity Disorder: Diagnosis and Management of ADHD in Children, Young People and Adults.* Clinical guidelines CG72. National Institute for Clinical and Health Excellence, London. http://guidance.nice.org.uk/ CG72.

Taylor, E. *et al.* (2004) European Clinical Guidelines for Hyperkinetic Disorder. *European Child and Adolescent Psychiatry* (suppl. 1), **13**, 1/7–1/30.

With thanks to Psychiatry at Medicine Publishing for their permission to allow adaptation of figures published in Bruce and Evans (2008).

CHAPTER 11

Learning disabilities

Angela Hassiotis and Martha Buszewicz

Case history

A 20-year-old man with mild learning disabilities and cerebral palsy has been attending his GP surgery for a while complaining of feeling unwell and that he 'sees faces in his breakfast cereal in the morning'. He appears to have neglected himself and to be confused. He admits to occasionally smoking cannabis. He lives by himself in a council flat and finds it difficult to cope. He has told his doctor that he heard voices telling him to harm himself.

The GP, following a mental state examination and a risk assessment, makes an urgent referral to the local community learning disabilities service asking for an assessment. The consultant psychiatrist and a community psychiatric nurse from the Community Learning Disabilities Team carry out a detailed assessment. He is diagnosed as suffering from a psychotic disorder and is commenced on antipsychotic medication. A deterioration in the patient's mental state necessitates further referral to the Crisis Team and a short period of intensive home treatment as an alternative to hospital admission. During this time the community team remain involved. The patient begins to show improvement and a meeting under the Care Programme Approach is convened. He continues to visit the practice for prescriptions. His care coordinator, the community psychiatric nurse, monitors his progress including adherence to antipsychotic medication, and side-effects (e.g. extrapyramidal symptoms), and liaises with other professionals to enhance his social support and with the GP for health surveillance.

Introduction

Primary healthcare is the cornerstone of care provision in the UK. General practitioners are expected to assess, investigate and manage a wide variety of health problems, often dealing with complex long-term conditions. People with learning disabilities (see Box 11.1) have increased health difficulties compared with the general population, but they may remain underrepresented within the primary care setting. This may be because they have problems accessing the service, or because their medical problems are not fully detected and dealt with when they do attend because of communication or other complexities.

Box 11.1 Definition of learning disability

Learning disability is a significant impairment of intellectual functioning (often measured using IQ tests), alongside a significant impairment of social/adaptive functioning, which is present from childhood. The International Classification of Diseases, tenth revision (ICD-10), divides learning disability into four categories: mild (IQ 50–69), moderate (IQ 35–49), severe (IQ 20–34), and profound (IQ less than 20).

A practice of approximately 7,500 patients will have 25 patients with learning disabilities registered (0.33%) whilst the prevalence of the spectrum of learning disabilities from mild to severe and profound is almost 3% of the entire population. Such discrepancy may be due to the fact that several individuals who have mild learning disabilities may not be identified and thus not known to specialist services. The Michael inquiry (2008) has highlighted the gaps in healthcare provision that people with learning disabilities receive and has called for improvements in the training and skills development of undergraduate medical students in order to meet the needs of this population group. A recent government initiative (Quality and Outcomes Framework) requires GPs to identify all registered patients with a learning disability on their lists. There is significant evidence that supports the effectiveness of health checks in reducing morbidity and mortality in people with learning disabilities. In the light of this information, in England, Primary Care Trusts (PCTs) are piloting the use of locally direct enhanced schemes (DESs) which require GPs to offer an annual health check and undertake awareness training amongst their practice staff, in addition to setting up and maintaining a register of patients with a learning disability.

Physical health problems

Common conditions that are seen in people with learning disabilities include sensory impairments (in up to 24% of cases) and epilepsy (35%), which may be poorly controlled in a significant minority of patients). Other conditions that are secondary to learning disabilities include obesity due to sedentary lifestyles, and in some cases the use of antipsychotic medications that can cause people to put on weight. Poor dental care, constipation and osteoporosis may also be associated with significant morbidity.

There are significant potential health inequalities affecting this population. These may be due to treatable medical conditions undiagnosed or left untreated (see above) and/or the poor uptake of health promotion such as smoking cessation services, which may be difficult for this group of people to access effectively (Kerr, 2006). Barriers to access or delivery of healthcare are shown in Box 11.2.

Box 11.2 Barriers to healthcare

- Mobility problems
- Mental disorders and problem behaviours
- Poor knowledge and skills of primary care staff
- Communication problems affecting uptake of available health care resources
- Lack of resources and insufficient time for consultation
- Poverty

Mental health disorders in people with learning disabilities

Learning disabilities are associated with increased psychiatric morbidity (Cooper *et al.*, 2007; point prevalence of mental disorders is shown in Table 11.1). In addition, certain genetic disorders present with both increased mental and physical health comorbidity; for example, people with Down's syndrome are more susceptible to heart defects, hypothyrodism and dementia of Alzheimer's type. People with Prader–Willi syndrome suffer with hypotonia, obesity and affective psychosis. Fragile X is linked with heart abnormalities, premature ovarian failure in female carriers, a neurological condition in older male

Table 11.1 Point prevalence rates of mental ill health as defined by clinical examination and DC-LD* diagnostic criteria (Cooper et al., 2007).

Diagnostic category	Clinical diagnosis (n = 1023) %	DC-LD diagnosis (n = 1023) %
Psychotic disorder	4.4	3.8
Affective disorder	6.6	5.7
Anxiety disorder	3.8	3.1
Obsessive compulsive disorder	0.7	0.5
Organic disorder	2.2	2.1
Alcohol/substance use disorder	1.0	0.8
Attention deficit hyperactivity disorder	1.5	1.2
Autistic spectrum disorder	7.5	4.4
Problem behaviour	22.5	18.7
Mental ill health of any type, excluding autistic spectrum disorder	37.0	32.8
Mental ill health of any type	40.9	35.2

*DC-LD: diagnostic criteria in Learning Disability

carriers (ataxia, memory loss and intention tremor) and finally hyperactivity and autism-like behaviours.

People with learning disabilities may have many causal factors for mental illness that include genetic vulnerability, substance misuse, multiple disabilities and physical illness, prescribed drug interactions, bullying, low self-esteem as a result of adverse life events and coping strategies, poverty, stigma and limited social networks, to name but a few (Cooper and Simpson, 2006).

Common mental disorders

Common mental disorders (depression and anxiety) have been shown to be 3 to 4 times more prevalent in people with mild learning disabilities and may account for almost 50% of the diagnoses of problem behaviours in those with severe learning disabilities.

Although the symptoms of depression are similar to the symptoms seen in the general population, more 'behaviour-based' symptoms may occur as service users may not know how to express their distress due to communication difficulties or more severe learning disabilities. The diagnosis of depression should be considered in the presence of self-injury, aggression, other destructive behaviours, loss of adaptive behaviour skills, reduced communication, social withdrawal, onset of or increase in problem behaviours, and reassurance-seeking behaviour. The GP needs to use informant observations in addition to self-report, and appreciate that people with learning disabilities who are significantly depressed may for example present with lower levels of energy, an increase in maladaptive behaviours and a significant increase in somatic complaints, rather than the more standard depressive symptoms of tearfulness, feeling guilty and poor concentration.

Symptoms of anxiety such as excessive worrying, avoidance of potentially feared stimuli, and physiological signs such as the feeling of choking and palpitations may not be reliably reported or may be misinterpreted and therefore anxiety disorders may be under-diagnosed in people with learning disabilities.

Psychosis

Psychosis, broadly defined, is at least three times more common in people with learning disabilities than in the general population. Cooper *et al.* (2007) found a prevalence rate of psychotic disorder of 5.8% in adults with mild intellectual disabilities and 3.5% in those with moderate to profound intellectual disabilities. Psychosis includes abnormalities in thought content and form, speech and behaviour. Psychotic illnesses can vary from a short-lived episode which resolves spontaneously, to a chronic disorder, such as schizophrenia. Psychosis may be diagnosed in people with mild learning disabilities, but it is accepted that it is more difficult to diagnose in those with severe learning disabilities due to a lack of verbal skills to describe symptoms (Hassiotis and Sinai, 2009).

Other complex disorders

Often individuals with learning disabilities may show additional problem behaviours (particularly aggression towards others), may neglect themselves and also have comorbid autistic spectrum disorders. On these occasions, the GP may be required to exclude any underlying physical problems that may account for the problem behaviours and consider appropriate interventions such as pain management or further referrals. The overall treatment of such conditions will be coordinated primarily by the local community learning disabilities service, but there may be occasions where shared care arrangements are necessary. For example, the GP will be involved in any follow-up prescribing and in the provision of overall healthcare to the service user. Very often the GP's viewpoint and assistance in monitoring those who engage poorly with services is invaluable.

Assessment of people with learning disabilities

In diagnosing a mental disorder the following must be taken into account:

- People with learning disability may be highly suggestible, so it is important to phrase questions carefully
- Delusions may be fleeting and be quite simple in content
- The person may be unable to describe symptoms, although they may clearly appear to experience symptoms such as hallucinations
- There may be a temporary exacerbation of problem behaviours or regression in skills

History taking

The assessment of mental disorder in people with learning disabilities should follow a similar pattern as in the general population, although there should be more emphasis on a developmental perspective and the social context. It is important to take a positive approach, emphasising the service user's abilities rather than disabilities. It is advisable to greet the person with learning disabilities before the carer, and communication should include accessible materials such as pictures and gestures or sign language, although the GP must first establish whether the person uses any such means. Problems in communication may stem from cognitive deficits in the person with learning disabilities, difference in symptom description by carers (e.g. agitation may be confused with aggression) and the skill of the interviewer.

The clinician should establish the current medication list and any investigations and procedures that might have already taken place.

The main components of assessing an individual with a learning disability are:

1. Assessment of the presenting complaint

Here it is important to gather information from observation (particularly if the person has poor verbal skills) or interview with the patient and collateral history from informants such as paid or family carers, with a specific focus on any changes noted in the patient's behaviour from his or her longstanding state. Collateral information is especially important, as people with learning disabilities may be unable to place events in their correct time frame or give the duration of illness.

2. Consideration of other health comorbidities is imperative

Additional sensory impairments or disorders such as epilepsy should be noted. The clinician will need to identify known problems or conditions that may be relevant to his or her current treatment and anything that may be linked to the service user's cause of disability (if known).

3. Investigations and referrals for specialist assessment should be made if needed

It is essential that the interpretation of findings from the assessment are embedded within a developmental context, as this approach may reduce the occurrence of 'diagnostic overshadowing', where the co-existing mental disorder is seen as a representation of the learning disability and thus may remain untreated.

The GP should formulate an appropriate plan of management that should be discussed with the person and their network, including other professionals who may be involved in his or her care.

When a GP is contacted out of hours for an urgent assessment where the presenting complaint is one of problem behaviours, it is particularly essential to weigh up the possibility of discomfort or other physical complaints before a psychiatric assessment is arranged or psychotropic medication prescribed. In addition, the person's developmental level should be taken into consideration, as it could explain the reasons behind the person's problem behaviours (e.g. head banging occurs at about 18 months of life; temper tantrums are seen at 2 to 3 years of age).

Differential diagnosis

Agitation, irritability, anxiety and lethargy may be the presenting symptoms of a number of disorders; therefore it is essential to consider other diagnostic possibilities especially as people with learning disabilities are likely to have comorbid conditions. The commonest differential diagnoses include:

- Physical illness
    - Epilepsy – in particular, temporal lobe epilepsy
    - Infection (e.g. urinary or respiratory tract infections, meningitis)
    - Hearing or visual impairment (e.g. hallucinations or illusions due to visual impairment can be seen in Charles Bonnet syndrome)

- Causes of pain or distress (e.g. toothache, earache, constipation or menstrual pain)
- Drug or alcohol related causes
  - Alcoholic hallucinosis or drug-induced psychosis
  - Sensitivity to prescribed medication
- Other psychiatric illness
  - Affective illness
  - Anxiety disorder
  - Dementia (e.g. visual hallucinations in Lewy-body dementia)
- Autistic spectrum disorders

Management

People with learning disabilities have a right to access generic services with additional input where required. If the GP suspects the presence of a mental health disorder, a referral to the community learning disabilities service should be made, although often GPs may commence treatment in uncomplicated cases. Sometimes admission to hospital may be required for further observation and to commence and establish treatment, particularly in cases of severe mental disorders or poor adherence. A risk assessment should also be conducted to ensure that the person is not at risk of harming him- or herself or the public. Where the patient has no insight and refuses voluntary admission the Mental Health Act 1983 may be applied so that he or she may be detained under section 2 (for assessment) or 3 (for assessment and/or treatment).

The treatment of mental disorders in people with learning disabilities follows similar principles to those used in the general population. Effective treatments include:

- Antipsychotic or antidepressant medication, but dosage must be tapered slowly according to response and to avoid exacerbation of epilepsy or side-effects (see Chapter 17 for more details). Accessible medication leaflets are available.
- Psychotherapeutic interventions; relaxation training; psychoeducation; desensitisation; and lately cognitive behavioural therapy. It should be noted that the latter is usually modified to take into account the cognitive limitations in this patient group; therefore sessions may be shorter and rely on accessible materials to enhance communication ability and concentration.
- Other therapies such as modified yoga and drama and music therapies have all been used with encouraging results (for details see http://apt.rcpsych.org/cgi/reprint/11/5/355.pdf).

■ The use of controlled multisensory environments, also called snoezelen (http://www.isna.de/index2e.html), may be helpful in calming and reducing stress in people with severe learning disabilities. Speech and language therapists may help to devise appropriate strategies for helping the individual during multisensory sessions. The NICE guidelines, though not specifically devised for this population, are applicable to a variety of interventions for mental health disorders.

When interventions such as physical examination, investigations and treatment are concerned, the person's consent is required, or if they lack capacity, a decision should be made in their best interests (see Chapter 15).

Despite the wide variation of community learning disabilities services across the UK, many community teams have access to specialist mental health services, such as Crisis Intervention, alternative facilities to hospital admission or rehabilitation services. The aim is to treat a person with learning disabilities wherever possible in their own home, with input from learning disabilities professionals. Social support is now provided through a combination of statutory services and personalised budgets, which allow greater flexibility and tailor-made care.

Learning disabilities service structure

Services are multidisciplinary and employ one or more professionals from a range of disciplines. GPs can usually refer directly to the community learning disabilities services by letter, telephone or email. All referrals are usually discussed in weekly team meetings and cases allocated to professionals for an initial assessment which helps to clarify the care pathway.

The learning disabilities services usually work together with other agencies (e.g. voluntary sector, education) in order to promote citizenship and equality for people with learning disabilities in the domains of health, housing, education and employment as described for England in *Valuing People Now* (Department of Health, 2009), the follow up document of the original White Paper *Valuing People* (http://valuingpeople.gov.uk/). These targets may be achieved through Person-Centred Plans, a Community Care Assessment to investigate accommodation, daytime activities and occupational needs, and finally a Carers' Assessment to identify problems associated with the caring role if the person resides with his or her family.

Key points

- Tailor communication level to the service user's ability and use accessible information to enhance the message.
- Mental health disorders may be caused by comorbid and undiagnosed physical illness.
- Treat any underlying psychiatric disorder and try to avoid non-specific treatment of problem behaviours, which may themselves be indicative of a physical or mental health problem.
- Use multiple informants where possible, and consider the person with learning disabilities in their social context.
- The treatment of mental disorders is similar to that in the general population, but drug doses should start low and be increased slowly due to greater risk of side-effects.

Further reading and bibliography

Cooper, S. A., Smiley, E., Morrison, J. *et al.* (2007) Mental ill health in adults with intellectual disability: prevalence and associated factors. *British Journal of Psychiatry*, **190**, 27–35.

Cooper, S. A. and Simpson, N. (2006) Assessment and classification of psychiatric disorders in adults with learning disabilities. *Psychiatry*, **5**, 306–11.

Department of Health (2009) *Valuing People Now*. DoH, London. http://www.dh.gov.uk/prod_consum_dh/groups/dh_digitalassets/documents/digitalasset/dh_093375.pdf . Accessed 16 July 2010.

Hassiotis, A. and Sinai, A. (2009) Psychosis. In: *Intellectual Disabilities Psychiatry: a Practical Guide* (eds. A. Hassiotis, D. Andrea Barron and I. Hall). Wiley, Chichester.

Michael, J. (2008) *Healthcare for All.* http://www.oldt.nhs.uk/documents/Healthcare-forall.pdf. Accessed 4 January 2010.

Kerr, M. (2006) Assessment in Primary Care. *Psychiatry*, **5**, 351–4.

CHAPTER 12

Mental health problems in the elderly

Joanne Rodda, Shirlony Morgan, Faye Dannhauser and Thomas Dannhauser

Case history 1

Mr A is a 72-year-old man who has had generally good health through-out his life. His hypertension is well controlled on medication and he had surgery for an inguinal hernia one year ago. After his operation he became very confused for a couple of days but seemed to recover.

His wife brings him to see his GP when she becomes concerned about his deteriorating memory. Around two years ago she started to notice that he was forgetting the names of friends he had not seen for a while. Since then he has become increasingly forgetful and often repeats himself in conversations, gets his grandchildren's names muddled and has some word-finding difficulties. He gets up and dressed in the morn-ing but needs a bit of prompting to find clean clothes. He used to pay all the household bills by post but his son has changed them to direct debit. Mr A insists that his memory is good for his age, but agrees to seeing the doctor if it makes Mrs A feel better. Mrs A asks if her concerns are justified and whether there is any treatment available for this type of problem.

Case history 2

Sixty-eight-year-old Mrs E goes to her GP for a routine review of her diabetic medication. He makes some general enquiries and finds out that Mrs E has been feeling tired and low in energy. She has stopped going to her regular social club and thinks this is because she has 'bad nerves'. She has lost 7 lb in weight and is not sleeping too well. Other than well-controlled type 2 diabetes and hypertension, Mrs E's past medical history is unremarkable.

Dementia

Dementia is common and will become more so as the elderly population grows. The prevalence in 60–64-year-olds is less than 1%, but increases with age so that more than 24% of the over 80s in the western world are affected. It is one of the main causes of disability in the elderly.

Dementia is an acquired impairment in multiple cognitive domains which is usually progressive and irreversible and occurs in the presence of clear consciousness. Alzheimer's disease is the most common cause of dementia and is responsible for 50–60% of cases. There are many causes of dementia and dementia-like syndromes (Table 12.1).

Investigation of cognitive impairment and diagnosis of dementia in the elderly is important in order to:

Table 12.1 Causes of dementia and dementia-like syndromes.

Cause	Examples
Neurodegenerative	Alzheimer's disease
	Dementia with Lewy bodies
	Parkinson's disease dementia
	Frontotemporal dementia
	Rarer diseases (e.g. Huntington's disease, Creutzfeldt–Jakob disease)
Vascular	Cerebrovascular disease
	Intracranial bleed (e.g. subdural haematoma)
Inflammatory/ autoimmune	Vasculitis
	Multiple sclerosis
Infective	Neurosyphilis, HIV
Trauma	Head injury
	Dementia pugalistica (Boxer's dementia)
Other	Metabolic/endocrine (e.g. hypothyroidism, renal failure)
	Vitamin deficiency (e.g. B12, folate, thiamine)
	Toxic (e.g. alcohol)
	Neoplastic
	Depression ('depressive pseudodementia')
	Normal pressure hydrocephalus

- Exclude and treat potentially reversible causes
- Provide appropriate treatment for the dementia
- Enable access to support services
- Identify the dementia subtype

Differentiating between different dementia subtypes is important because of differences in the natural course of the disease and response to treatment. For example, cholinesterase inhibitors are prescribed in Alzheimer's disease but have little benefit in frontotemporal dementia. In dementia with Lewy bodies, use of antipsychotic medication may lead to severe adverse drug reactions. The identification of cerebrovascular disease highlights the need for modification of vascular risk factors. Awareness of the likely progression of a person's dementia subtype can help them and their families to have an idea of what to expect in the future and to prepare for this both practically and psychologically.

Clinical features

Alzheimer's disease

- Characterised by gradual onset and slow progression
- Initial deficits in short-term memory
- Language deficits, e.g. nominal dysphasia (word-finding problems) are common and more gross difficulties develop later
- Agnosia and apraxia are also common, especially later in the disease
- Median survival from diagnosis is six years

Onset below the age of 65 is unusual and is sometimes associated with an inherited (autosomal dominant) form of the disease

Vascular dementia

- A wide variety of presentations exist which can include the following features: sudden onset; stepwise progression; focal neurological symptoms and signs; patchy cognitive deficits; relative sparing of short-term memory; and emotional lability
- May occur as a result of pathology ranging from a single strategic infarct to widespread small vessel ischaemia

- Vascular risk factors are important, but not diagnostic
- Neuroimaging is often helpful for diagnosis (Box 12.1)
- Average survival is five years from onset and approximately 50% of patients die from ischaemic heart disease
- Comorbidity with Alzheimer's or other neurodegenerative pathology is common

---

Box 12.1 Investigation of dementia in primary and secondary care (adapted from NICE guidelines (2006))

Primary care
- Full blood count, creatinine/urea and electrolytes, liver function tests, calcium, glucose, thyroid function tests, serum B12 and folate, lipid profile
- Investigations to rule out delirium, e.g. midstream urine testing or chest X-ray if indicated

Secondary care
- Structural neuroimaging (MRI preferable)
- HMPAO SPECT or FDG PET (perfusion scan) if diagnosis of Alzheimer's disease, FTD or vascular dementia is difficult to differentiate
- FP-CIT SPECT scanning if suspected DLB but diagnosis is difficult to establish

Not recommended as routine
- Syphilis serology, HIV testing, CSF studies, EEG

Dementia with Lewy bodies (DLB)

- The central feature is progressive cognitive decline that interferes with normal function
- Core features are fluctuations in attention and cognition, visual hallucinations and spontaneous motor symptoms of Parkinson's disease
- Other features include sensitivity to antipsychotic drugs, falls, autonomic instability and REM sleep behaviour disorder ('acting out' of dreams due to loss of muscle atonia during sleep)

■ DLB and dementia in Parkinson's disease form part of the same spectrum of disorders associated with Lewy body pathology; differentiation is based arbitrarily on the timing of onset of motor and cognitive symptoms

Frontotemporal dementia (FTD)

■ Umbrella term for a group of neurodegenerative conditions that affect the frontal and/or temporal lobes
■ Patients can present with behavioural or language variants
■ There are several types of underlying pathology (NB Pick's disease is a well-known cause of FTD, but is in fact quite rare)
■ The age of onset is between 45 and 65 years but can occur at any stage in adulthood
■ Onset is insidious and progression gradual
■ Core features include early impairment in social and personal conduct with emotional blunting and loss of insight
■ FTD is associated with a wide variety of behavioural and speech abnormalities (e.g. perseveration, stereotypies, echolalia, mental rigidity and inflexibility, hyperorality) as well as physical signs (e.g. primitive reflexes, incontinence and Parkinsonian symptoms)

Differentiating between types of dementia

The overlap in symptomatology between different types of dementia means that accurate diagnosis is not always straightforward. Comorbid pathology may also complicate diagnosis, and over 50% of patients with dementia have multiple types of potentially causative neuropathology identifiable at autopsy. At present, the majority of patients with dementia are given a single diagnosis representing the most likely underlying disease process. In the future, advances in neuroimaging and other diagnostic techniques may allow more accurate diagnosis of multiple dementia subtypes.

Mild Cognitive Impairment (MCI)

In MCI there are objective cognitive deficits, but activities of daily living are preserved and criteria for diagnosis of dementia are not met. People with MCI are at an increased risk of dementia and the conversion rate of the amnestic type (aMCI) is reported to be 10–15% per year. However, definitions, diagnosis and investigation of MCI vary between treatment centres and there is still considerable debate about the concept.

Assessment

This includes: a detailed history (including informant history where possible); medication review; cognitive and mental state examination; physical examination and appropriate investigations (see Box 12.1). Early exclusion of delirium and treatment of the underlying cause (e.g. urinary tract infection, chest infection, constipation) is important and referral to specialist services should not be allowed to delay this; longer episodes of untreated delirium are associated with poorer outcomes. Patients with dementia are particularly susceptible to delirium and the two conditions often coexist. Table 12.2 summarises the differences in presentation between delirium and dementia.

There are several tools that can be used for brief cognitive testing. The Mini-Mental State Examination is perhaps the best known, although there are other options which have been developed for use within the primary care setting, including the 6-item Cognitive Impairment Test (6-CIT), the General Practitioner Assessment of Cognition (GPCOG) and the 7-Minute Screen. The 6-CIT (Box 12.2) is a useful test that can be easily used in the primary care setting. As a screening tool for dementia, it has comparable specificity and higher sensitivity than the MMSE.

It is important to take into account any factors which may affect performance on these tests, for example sensory impairment, educational level, language, physical illness and depression.

Table 12.2 Clinical features of delirium and dementia.

Characteristic	Delirium	Dementia
Onset	Acute	Insidious
Duration	Transient	Chronic
Course	Fluctuating	Progressive
Attention	Reduced	Intact initially
Consciousness	Altered	Normal
Hallucinations	Common	Less common

Box 12.2 The 6-item Cognitive Impairment Test (6-CIT)

	Max. error	Score	Weight		Weighted score
1. What year is it?	1	____	× 4	=	____
2. What month is it now?	1	____	× 3	=	____
	Memory phrase – Ask the patient to repeat an address after you for later recall:				
	John/Brown/42/West/Street/Bedford				
3. About what time is it (within 1 hr)?	1	____	× 3	=	____
4. Count backwards from 20 to 1	2	____	× 2	=	____
5. Say the months in reverse order	2	____	× 2	=	____
6. Repeat the memory phrase	5	____	× 2	=	____
	TOTAL				____

NB: One point is given for each **incorrect** response (maximum points for errors on each item is specified); this is then multiplied by the weighting for that item to give a weighted score. Weighted scores are added to give total out of 28. A score of ≥ 8 suggests dementia (sensitivity 90%, specificity 100%; less sensitive in mild dementia (78%))

Referring to specialist services

In a patient presenting with cognitive decline, have a low threshold for referral to secondary care once reversible causes have been ruled out. If in doubt about contributions from physical illness or psychosocial stress, it may be worth arranging to see the patient again before referring.

A detailed referral from the GP will assist specialist services in determining the most appropriate initial contact (e.g. initial assessment of risk by community mental health worker, domiciliary visit by psychiatrist, outpatient clinic, specialist memory clinic etc.) and the degree of urgency. Points to highlight in the referral are:

- Onset and nature of cognitive symptoms
- Behavioural disturbances

- Impact on activities of daily living, social activity, relationships
- Risks to self (e.g. neglect, exploitation, vulnerability, wandering)
- Risks to others (e.g. aggression)
- Current level of support, e.g. family support, care package details
- Previous contact with psychiatric services
- Medical history and current medication
- Contact details for an informant
- Other professionals involved
- Investigations undertaken to rule out reversible cause

Management

The management of dementia relies on integration of primary and secondary health care and social services.

Drug treatment of dementia

The use of cholinesterase inhibitors (donepezil, rivastigmine and galantamine) is sanctioned by NICE (2006) for the management of the cognitive symptoms of Alzheimer's disease of moderate severity and in the management of 'behaviour that challenges' in Alzheimer's disease and DLB under certain circumstances (see Box 12.3). These guidelines have been associated with significant controversy, and clinical practice varies between centres. There is also convincing evidence for the use of cholinesterase inhibitors for cognitive symptoms in DLB. Many Primary Care Trusts have protocols for shared care with respect to ongoing monitoring and prescription of these medications.

The most common side-effects of cholinesterase inhibitors are diarrhoea and nausea/vomiting. These usually pass within two weeks, although they can be severe enough to necessitate stopping the drug. Starting at a low dose and titrating gradually minimises the risks of these problems. The main caution is bradycardia or heart block, and an ECG or cardiology opinion may be requested in some cases. Other cautions include history of upper GI bleed, epilepsy and COPD/asthma.

Memantine is an NMDA receptor antagonist and is licensed for use in moderate to severe dementia in Alzheimer's disease. Use in clinical practice is not recommended in the 2006 NICE guidance; therefore prescription will depend on individual specialist practice and will usually be on an individual named-patient basis.

Box 12.3 Summary of current NICE guidance for use of cholinesterase inhibitors in dementia

Alzheimer's disease
- Drugs recommended are donepezil, rivastigmine, galantamine.
- For cognitive symptoms in moderately severe dementia.
- Treatment may only be initiated by specialists.
- Six-monthly review of MMSE score, behaviour and global functioning. Can be conducted in primary care if local shared care protocol in place.
- For severe non-cognitive symptoms where non-pharmacological treatment and antipsychotic drugs have been unsuccessful or inappropriate (in mild, moderate or severe dementia).

Other types of dementia
- Non-cognitive symptoms of DLB (no mention of use for cognitive symptoms of DLB).
- Not recommended in vascular dementia.
- Not recommended for use in mild cognitive impairment.

Support for carers

An assessment of the needs of carers should form part of the care plan put in place by specialist services. Carers may benefit from peer-group support, psychoeducation and practical support in the form of respite care or sitting services. Admiral Nurses are specialist mental health nurses working within the NHS to support the families of people with dementia, and are supported by the national charity Dementia UK. This charity has several other branches of support for the carers and families of people with dementia (http://www.dementiauk.org/what-we-do/admiral-nurses/). Other voluntary sector organisations include the Alzheimer's Society (http://alzheimers.org.uk/) and Age Concern.

Dementia and driving

A diagnosis of dementia does not automatically mean that a person will have their licence revoked, but a person with dementia is obliged by law to inform the DVLA of their diagnosis if they wish to continue to drive. The DVLA will then usually request information from their GP or specialist doctor and may arrange an assessment of the person's fitness to drive. If it becomes known to a doctor that a patient with dementia is continuing to drive without having informed the DVLA it is their duty to do so themselves.

End of life care in dementia

Dementia accounts for one in three deaths in an average general practice and is usually the result of physical illness associated with older age. However, for some, survival into the late stages of dementia can result in high levels of distress and disability in the final weeks or months of life, and the need for complex management and ethical decisions.

Good end of life care in dementia is essentially palliative care, and the goal is to alleviate suffering rather than to prolong life. Patients with severe dementia may not be able to communicate the cause of their distress, which may be due to pain, constipation, incontinence, vulnerable pressure areas, immobility or other factors. Eating and drinking in patients with end-stage dementia is an emotive issue; the normal mechanisms of thirst and hunger are disrupted and there may be mechanical difficulties with chewing and swallowing. This may cause more distress for carers and healthcare professionals than for the patient themselves, and PEG or NG tube feeding is controversial. In general, decisions are made in consultation with the family, but in the UK the general view is that this is rarely in the best interests of the patient.

Management of symptoms in the end stages of dementia may require medication in some instances, for example for agitation and pain. This should ideally be integrated with other strategies aimed at relieving distress, including psychological and spiritual approaches. Massage, physiotherapy, pressure relief and aromatherapy may be effective although not always available (see Table 12.3).

Behavioural and psychological symptoms of dementia (BPSD)

The term BPSD encompasses a broad range of symptoms and signs, including agitation, aggression, apathy, mood changes, wandering, disinhibition, sleep disturbance, hallucinations and delusions. These symptoms are often perceived by care-givers as more distressing than the cognitive symptoms of dementia and are associated with an earlier move to institutional care.

Table 12.3 General principles of management of dementia.

Management	Characteristics
Functional	Occupational therapy assessment; maximise level of independence with activities of daily living; environmental modifications
Social	Accommodation to suit needs, social care package, telecare, meals on wheels, financial and legal issues (e.g. lasting power of attorney etc.), structured activities (e.g. day centre)
Risk	Identify and minimise risks, for example neglect, vulnerability, gas taps etc.
Pharmacological treatment	May be appropriate for management of cognitive and/ or behavioural symptoms
Psychological treatment	Psychological interventions including reminiscence, music, art and behavioural therapies may be of benefit
Carer support	Education, involvement in decision making, psychological support (e.g. carers groups, voluntary sector organisations), respite care
Physical health needs	Treatment of comorbid physical illness, liaison with between primary and secondary care and between specialist teams

BPSD may be due to many factors, including:

- changes in environment, routine or care staff
- pain, constipation, medication side-effects or any underlying acute or chronic physical illnesses (e.g. urinary tract and chest infections, heart failure, COPD and poorly controlled diabetes)
- progression of underlying neurodegenerative disease

The most important part of the assessment and management of behavioural disturbance in dementia is the identification and treatment of any potentially reversible causes. Interventions directed towards the behaviour itself may involve modification of the environment, daily routine or approach of care staff towards the patient. In complex cases, input from secondary care psychology or mental health nursing staff may be appropriate. NICE guidance (2006) advocates the use of aromatherapy, multi-sensory stimulation, massage, music, dancing and animal therapy. Given the often limited availability of these therapies, medication is often used (see Table 12.4). Evidence for the efficacy of any medication in the management of BPSD is limited and potential benefits

Box 12.4 Risks associated with use of antipsychotic medications for behavioural and psychological symptoms of dementia (BPSD)

The Committee on Safety of Medicines (CSM) issued a statement in 2004 regarding the increased risk of stroke with risperidone and olanzapine in dementia. This was based on pooled data from several RCTs. Soon after, the United States Food and Drug Administration issued a statement regarding increased mortality when atypical antipsychotic drugs were used in dementia. More recent evidence and warnings have highlighted safety concerns regarding both typical and atypical antipsychotic drugs. Other adverse effects include movement disorder, postural hypotension, constipation and increased confusion. Use of antipsychotic drugs in BPSD is therefore a compromise between the need for symptom control and the potential adverse effects. If it is necessary to use these drugs, use should be limited to 12 weeks whilst alternative approaches are explored.

must be balanced against the risk of side-effects. Most evidence exists for risperidone and olanzapine but both drugs are associated with an increased risk of mortality and stroke (see Box 12.4).

Depression

Prevalence estimates of depression in the elderly vary widely depending on the setting and the diagnostic criteria. Although age in itself is not a risk factor for depression, many risk factors for depression are associated with age, for example physical illness, disability and bereavement.

Presentation

Older people may be less likely to describe feelings of sadness and low mood, and there can be confusion between symptoms of depression and those of physical illness (e.g. chronic pain, apathy, fatigue and disability). Symptoms

Table 12.4 Pharmacotherapy in BPSD.

Drug	Comments
Antipsychotics	Most widely used although often not justified. May be helpful in severe agitation and aggression or for psychotic symptoms. Most evidence is for risperidone (0.5–2 mg). Options with potentially fewer side-effects include quetiapine (25–200 mg) and aripiprazole (5–15 mg). Use should be ideally limited to a maximum of 12 weeks due to lack of evidence of efficacy in long-term use and risk of serious adverse events
Benzodiazepines	For short-term use lorazepam (start at 0.5 mg doses). Diazepam is longer-acting (start at 2 mg doses). Risks include tolerance, dependence, increased confusion and excessive sedation
Clomethiazole	Start at 1–2 capsules daily, can be increased. Also associated with tolerance, dependence, increased confusion and excessive sedation
Antidepressants	If depressive symptoms are present, consider citalopram (20 mg), trazodone (50–100 mg) or mirtazapine (15–45 mg, especially if concerns regarding appetite and sleep)
Anti-epileptic drugs	Carbamazepine (50–300 mg) and sodium valproate (250 mg – 1 g) may be helpful in agitation or aggression, although would usually be started in specialist practice
Cholinesterase inhibitors*	Evidence for modest effect on BPSD in Alzheimer's disease. May improve hallucinations in dementia with Lewy bodies
Memantine*	May be helpful for BPSD in Alzheimer's disease, particularly agitation

Suggested daily doses are given in the table; initially medication should be prescribed at the lower end of the range with slow titration as necessary.
*Prescribed in specialist setting

of depression and anxiety often co-exist in the elderly and it may be easier for older people to describe feeling anxious than feeling low or sad.

Depression may also be difficult to disentangle from dementia. Depression is a risk factor for dementia, and may also occur as part of the prodromal phase of dementia. Depression is also common in people with dementia, and some features of dementia like apathy and sleep–wake cycle disturbances can be confused with depressive symptomatology. Cognitive impairment resembling dementia may occur in depression at any age ('depressive pseudodementia'), but is more common in the elderly. The cognitive deficits resolve on treatment of depression, although these individuals are at high risk of developing dementia over the following years.

Where physical illness and cognitive impairment cloud the picture, it can be difficult to be clear of the diagnosis. The presence of biological features of depression, particularly diurnal mood variation, poor appetite, early morning waking and anhedonia are useful in making the distinction, as are feelings of guilt, helplessness and worthlessness.

Passive suicidal ideation in depression in the elderly is not uncommon, but suicidal acts and active thoughts of suicide must be taken seriously and referred to specialist services. The elderly form the highest risk group for completed suicide and of all age groups are most likely to die from a suicide attempt.

Bereavement is a factor which is particularly relevant to depression in the elderly. Grief shares many similarities with depression, and it is important not to 'medicalise' this process. However, a depressive episode may be triggered by a bereavement and it is equally important that this does not go unrecognised and untreated (see Box 12.5). Bereavement counselling should be accessible in primary care and may be helpful for many individuals, whether depression is present or not.

Management

The management of depression in older adults follows the same principles as in younger adults (see Chapter 2). SSRIs are generally first-line pharmacological therapy because of their relatively safe side-effect profile. Citalopram is a safe option with relatively little potential for interaction and is also one of the safest choices in most medical conditions, including hepatic and renal impairment and heart failure (refer to prescribing guidelines for dose recommendations). The use of tricyclics as first line treatment (e.g. amitriptylline, dosulepin etc.)

Box 12.5 Features suggestive of depressive illness in the context of bereavement

- Prominent feelings of worthlessness or guilt not related to the death of the loved one
- Suicidal ideation other than thoughts of being with the deceased
- Psychomotor retardation
- Prolonged or marked functional impairment
- Hallucinations other than the image or voice of the loved one
- Prolonged grief (≥ 6 months)

is unwise given the side-effect profile and the availability of better alternatives. Use of low doses of amitriptyline as a night sedative is not justified.

Older people should not be maintained on sub-therapeutic doses of antidepressant medication (e.g. citalopram 10 mg, amitriptyline 25 mg) unless there has clearly been a maximal response. If a medication is not effective or cannot be successfully titrated upwards due to side-effects, an alternative should be prescribed where a therapeutic dose is tolerated (e.g. mirtazapine or duloxetine if an SSRI is not tolerated). In general, the lower limits of maintenance doses are the same in older and younger adults.

The therapeutic response may take as long as six weeks to be reached in the elderly, who are also at higher risk of relapse when medication is stopped. Longer or even indefinite periods of treatment may be necessary.

Psychological therapies including cognitive behavioural therapy are effective in older adults and should be considered as an alternative or adjunct to drug treatment in sub-threshold, mild or moderate depression. This type of therapy may be accessible within the primary care setting. In dementia or cognitive impairment, reminiscence therapy or behavioural therapy may be more appropriate, which may be accessible only via specialist psychiatry services.

Anxiety disorders

Anxiety is common in the elderly and often co-exists with depression. The most common anxiety disorder in old age is generalised anxiety disorder. Onset of panic disorder, phobias or obsessive compulsive disorder in old age is unusual.

In general, anxiety can be managed in primary care. As in younger adults, psychological therapy is usually the ideal first line management strategy. If pharmacological treatment is necessary, SSRIs are the first choice. Pregabalin is licensed for the treatment of generalised anxiety disorder. Benzodiazepines should be used with caution, ideally as a short-term measure, if symptoms are severe enough to warrant their use. Falls and confusion are a particular concern with these drugs, and tolerance and dependence may occur. If symptoms are refractive or particularly severe, referral to specialist psychiatric services is appropriate.

Bipolar affective disorder

The clinical features of mania in old age do not differ markedly from those in younger adults. However, first episode mania in old age is rare, and it is important that any underlying organic cause is excluded promptly. All individuals with hypomania or mania should be referred to specialist services. If mania is secondary to organic disorder, specialist advice from a psychiatrist on symptomatic treatment is often helpful.

First-line treatment of the acute symptoms of mania, whether primary or secondary, is with antipsychotic medication (e.g. olanzapine 5–10 mg, risperidone 1–2 mg, quetiapine 50–200 mg). Maintenance treatment with antipsychotic medication, lithium or sodium valproate is usually necessary and will normally be established by specialist services; monitoring of these medications may continue in primary care after a prolonged period of stability. In general, the target plasma level for lithium in the elderly is towards the lower end of the therapeutic window because the risk of toxicity is higher in this group. Monitoring of thyroid function and urea and electrolytes is also required.

Psychosis

The elderly population will include a proportion of individuals with life-long psychotic illness. As with mania, new onset of a primary psychotic illness in old age is unusual and an organic cause should be suspected and excluded. Urgent attention must be directed at excluding any reversible cause and early referral to psychiatry if none is found.

The terminology surrounding schizophrenia-like illnesses with an onset in late life is varied. Consensus terms are 'late-onset schizophrenia' if onset is between 40 and 60 years old and 'very late-onset schizophrenia-like psychosis' (VLOSLP) for the over-60s. Risk factors for VLOSLP include female gender, sensory impairment, social isolation and abnormal premorbid personality. VLOSLP is associated with hallucinations in any modality and delusions

---

Box 12.6 Causes of psychotic symptoms in the elderly

- Primary psychotic illness (e.g. schizophrenia, schizoaffective disorder, very late-onset schizophrenia-like psychosis, delusional disorder)
- Psychosis secondary to general medical conditions or drugs
- Depression or mania with psychotic features
- Dementia
- Sensory impairment (e.g. Charles Bonnet syndrome)

are usually systematised and persecutory; thought disorder and negative symptoms are uncommon.

Determining the cause of psychotic symptoms in old age is not always easy (Box 12.6). Before making a referral to specialist psychiatry services, it is important to try to understand the cause of the hallucinations or delusions, as failure to do so may result in unnecessary delays in treatment.

Management

- All individuals with a possible psychotic illness should be referred to specialist psychiatry services; reasonable efforts should be made to exclude an organic basis
- Pharmacological treatment is with antipsychotic drugs; doses may only need to be 1/10th of those used in younger adults
- Optimise hearing and vision by use of appropriate aids
- Psychological therapy, social support or admission to hospital may be necessary

Key points

- Have a low threshold for referring people with possible cognitive impairment for further assessment.
- Rule out delirium urgently in acute presentations of cognitive impairment and in behavioural disturbance in dementia.
- End of life care in dementia is essentially palliative care.
- Older people with depression need therapeutic doses of antidepressants, often take longer to respond and may need long-term maintenance therapy.
- All patients with a suspected primary manic or psychotic illness should be urgently referred to specialist services.

Further reading and bibliography

Alexopoulos, G. S. (2005) Depression in the elderly. *Lancet*, **365**, 1961–70.
Jolley, D., Hughes, J., Greaves, I., Jordan, A. and Sampson, E. (2008) Seeing patients with dementia through to the end of life. *Geriatric Medicine*, **38**, 461–4.

Khouzam, H. R., Battista, M. A., Emes, R. and Ahles, S. (2005) Psychosis in late life: evaluation and management of disorders seen in primary care. *Geriatrics*, **60**, 26–33.

NICE (2006) *Supporting People with Dementia and Their Carers in Health and Social Care*. Clinical guidelines CG42. National Institute of Clinical and Health Excellence, London. http://guidance.nice.org.uk/CG42.

Wetherell, J. L., Lenze, E. J. and Stanley, M. A. (2005) Evidence-based treatment of geriatric anxiety disorders. *Psychiatric Clinics of North America*, **28**, 871–96.

CHAPTER 13

Community mental health services for adults

Karl Marlowe and Gary Marlowe

Case history

A 22-year-old married Bangladeshi woman with a 10-month-old daughter came to the UK two years ago. The primary care team are concerned because she has recently expressed the belief that her neighbour is performing black magic. She has beliefs of spirit possession (jinn). Her father may have had similar problems but died a long time ago. She and her husband only want her to be seen by practising Islamic female staff.

- What services are available to provide an assessment?
- When is it appropriate to make a referral?
- How does one deal with the cultural issues and foster a therapeutic alliance?

Introduction

This chapter will discuss and describe the new community mental health services which are now routinely found all across the UK, and which were initially provided as a result of the National Service Framework (NSF) for mental health services launched in 1999. The subsequent policy drivers for mental health services and the service developments that followed are summarised in Table 13.1. Secondary care services are increasingly encouraged to align themselves with patients outside of the walls of large and impersonal hospitals. The developments in psychiatric services over the last decade have led to

Table 13.1 Policy drivers for mental health service reform in England (10 years).

Central DH policy	Overview	Outcomes
The NHS Plan (2000)	Extending the role of non-medical staff. To improve access and waiting time. To improve the knowledge and skill of NHS staff with new contracts of employment. To allow the private sectors to provide and become involved in services provision. To have a 'patient led' NHS. A clinical focus with new monies for Cancer, Heart Disease and Mental Health.	■ New contract for nurses, GP and consultant ■ Commissioning via PCTs ■ Primary care capital investment and PFI ■ Non-medical prescribers and clinical governance within NWW ■ DH published Policy Implementation Guidelines (PIG) for the new community mental health services.
The Mental Health Policy Implementation Guide (2001) (PIG) *Implementation of the National Service Framework (NSF) for Mental Health (1999)*	Describes how the NSF is to be achieved The PIG had a timeline, the service aims, the make-up of the team, its operational procedures and the targets for achievements at each phase of development. Described New Ways of Working with new staff at the Primary Care interface and mental health promotion	■ Three community teams: EIS, AOT, CRHTT ■ A commitment to have Mental Health Workers in Primary Care (counsellors) and in Secondary Care (gateway workers) ■ PCTs have a remit for mental health promotion. Integration of social and health care. Consideration of physical with mental health together
Our Health Our Care Our Say: a new direction for community services (2006)	Improving access to services, especially those who a socially marginalised and disadvantaged. This is of particular importance to Primary Care	■ Improving Access to Psychological Therapies (IAPT) commissioning toolkit (2008). For 1000s of CBT counsellors to be trained
High Quality Care for Everyone (2008)	Reference to a new NHS Constitution. Enable local priorities commissioned. Waiting time and access to GPs remain a commitment. Emphasis on clinical leadership, subsidiary, co-production for services and enabling NHS innovation	■ Improving social inclusion with Delivering Race Equality. Quality markers and performance reports ■ Early Intervention (including Child and adolescents) in mental health and Learning Disability a priority
New Horizons (2009)	To continue to focus on community services with an emphasis on early intervention/prevention and on improving access to difficult to reach communities	■ An extension of PIG for targets for new cases and for the effectiveness of the intervention provided by each service

DH = Department of Health; NHS = National Health Service; PCT = Primary Care Trust; NWW = New Ways of Working; IAPT = Improving Access to Psychological Therapies; EIS = Early Intervention Service; AOT = Assertive Outreach Team; CRHTT = Crisis Resolution and Home Treatment Team; PCT = Primary Care Trust: CBT = Cognitive behavioural therapy

a whole plethora of new acronyms, and it is hoped that these will make sense, both in definition and purpose, by the end of the chapter. Planning the patient care pathway for the case vignette will also be easier to navigate.

Community Mental Health Services

The new teams to deliver the NSF (1999) were Crisis Resolution, Assertive Outreach and Early Intervention. The evidence at the time for the proposals came from some preliminary research. However, there is little substantive evidence and no specific National Institute for Clinical Excellence (NICE) guidelines on mental health service models.

The policy to enhance community mental health services is aligned to the changes introduced by the Mental Health Act (2007), including Supervised Community Treatment Orders and a wider range of mental health professionals able to act as Responsible Clinicians (once the preserve of psychiatrists). A consequence of the NSF teams and New Ways of Working (NWW) has been the development of functional inpatient and functional community psychiatrists, with attendant further fragmentation (see Table 13.2).

Crisis Resolution/Home Treatment Team (CRHTT)

These teams aim to treat patents during an acute episode in the least restrictive environment practicable and as an alternative to hospital inpatient care. Referrals can come from primary care, Emergency Departments, CMHTs, inpatient teams, and (in some teams) direct service user and family referrals. These teams are sometimes split further into functional units with a Home Treatment Team (HTT) and a Crisis Team, which may be clinic based.

The interventions are intensive and may be more than once a day. They are time-limited and involve rapid assessment of the patient and their carer/family, medication monitoring, and risk assessment. They link appropriate social and health care, and a plan to avert further crisis, which may include advance directives in case the patient loses capacity. Home Treatment Teams are also involved in the facilitation of leave and discharge from hospitals. The CRHTTs are expected to have 14–16 staff serving a population of 150,000 and have between 20 and 30 patients on the caseload at any one time. CRHTTs have been tasked to develop day care or crisis homes/hostels. This is one of the areas for future service development. There is no doubt that CRHTTs have decreased the use of inpatient beds, but the new ways of working and positive risk taking raises the question of reduced continuity of care, associated increased morbidity for patients and disrupted historical and interpersonal communication with primary care teams

Assertive Outreach Team (AOT)

These teams aim to work with patients with severe and persistent mental disorders (e.g. schizophrenia and major affective disorders). Working age adults from aged 18 and up, who over a two-year period have high inpatient use (more than two admissions, or more than six months' hospitalisation, or Mental Health Act use) are deemed to be suitable. These patients would be expected to have functional disabilities, problems with engagement and have complex needs (violence, self-harm, vulnerability, substance misuse, depression or anxiety). The AOT model developed from an American study, the Program of Assertive Community Treatment (PACT), which showed some evidence of cost-effectiveness, improved engagement and reduced bed-days (Stein and Santos, 1998).

Assertive outreach provides continuity of care, with all staff involved in knowing and working with all patients. There is clinical leadership provided by a consultant psychiatrist, who would be expected to have a weekly clinical review meeting and provide oversight for all the multidisciplinary team members (Box 13.1).

The team would be expected to have 12–14 staff serving a population of 250,000, with each care coordinator having an allocation of 10–12 patients. The total caseload is expected to be on average 90 patients, but for inner city urban settings this could be substantially increased. Only secondary care mental health referrals are accepted. The more recent evidence shows a risk of high staff burnout and the questions of true functional recovery and cost effectiveness continue.

Early Intervention Service (EIS)

These teams aim to work with those aged 14–35 years old who have had their first episode of a schizophrenic disorder, with a time-limited duration of three

---

Box 13.1 Interventions provided by AOT

- Assessment of family/carer and cultural needs
- Proactive engagement and monitoring
- Medication administration and compliance
- Integrating work for comorbidity (e.g. addictions)
- Emphasis on basic daily living skills
- Rebuilding social networks
- Enabling functional recovery to stable mental health

years. The aim of an Early Intervention Service is of both a public health role by raising the awareness of schizophrenia, as well as providing clinical intervention. There is acknowledgement of diagnostic uncertainty, so the diagnosis 'schizophrenia' is replaced by the term 'psychosis', but the policy guidance is based on schizophrenia research (including the epidemiology on which the staff numbers and case load is based).

Early intervention teams are expected to see those in the acute phase of schizophrenia, by being proactive in detection and being rapid and flexible in assessments. They aim to treat in the least restrictive community setting, with a full assessment, including cultural and family needs. The interventions are dependent on the phase of the disorder and are evidenced by NICE guidelines for schizophrenia (2002, updated 2009). There is an expectation for antipsychotic medication to be started early and to reduce the Duration of Untreated Psychosis (DUP) and hence improve outcomes, including rates of relapse and physical, social and legal harm. During the recovery phase the intervention shifts to work on a shared explanatory model, family work on behaviour and psychoeducation, coping strategies for persistent symptoms and formalised cognitive behavioural therapy for certain patients. As with the Assertive Outreach model of care, the team should be integrated to treat comorbidity.

The policy guidance describes a service for a population of 1 million having 150 new cases per year and a caseload of 450 at full operation. In practice most Early Intervention teams are a third of this size and have 50 new cases per year and a caseload of 120–150, for a population of 250,000 to 300,000. There are on average 12–15 staff, with each care coordinator working with 15 patients. The recent evidence shows that Early Intervention may reduce the Duration of Untreated Psychosis and improve engagement, but not reduce the rate of relapse. The issue of diagnosis remains, as many teams do not restrict the service to a true first episode of schizophrenia and many teams do not have capacity to do rapid assessments or provide intervention, as they may have expanded too rapidly to fulfil a national caseload target.

Other mental health teams with a primary care interface

A number of other specialist mental health teams (see Table 13.2) have developed alongside the NSF teams, and all attempt to reduce the inpatient mental health service need. The Perinatal Psychiatric Services have been driven by repeated tragic deaths (maternal mental health is the primary cause of death for women in the first year after giving birth) sometimes involving a very young child. This is the only community mental health service which may lead to greater bed use, as there is very low tolerance for risk-taking. There is a proliferation of Community Rehabilitation Teams, often re-branded as Recovery

Table 13.2 Other community mental health developments (excluding Community Mental Health Teams (CMHTs)).

Teams	Pathway	Intervention
Personality disorders	Mainly secondary mental health services. Developing referrals from GP and Primary Care IAPT teams	Working on therapeutic communities, patient led. Using dialectic behaviour therapy and group psychodynamic therapy insights
Perinatal psychiatric	Primary care, midwives, obstetricians, CMHT and secondary mental health services	Expert assessments, close involvement with birth planning, advice for admission to Mother & Baby Mental Health Units. Risk assessment of the impact of maternal psychiatric morbidity during the 1 year post partum
Dual diagnosis	Primary care (including third sector organisations), CMHTs, CRHTT	Provide assessment within an assertive model to manage care during initial period. Start and advise treatment for both diagnoses. To provide training to a wide range of primary and secondary care settings
Community rehabilitation	Secondary care EIS, CMHT, wards for patients with persistent symptoms	Working with complex care with a 'recovery model' for functional recovery and rehabilitation
Improving Access to Psychological Therapies (IAPT)	Placed in primary care settings, as the majority of patients with depression/anxiety do not require secondary mental healthcare	Providing a stepped approach to the treatment for depression and for anxiety disorders with the provision of CBT (NICE guidelines). To encourage vocational and work by decreasing dependence on state benefits

Teams, to service the increased numbers of patients with chronic psychiatric disorders living in community supported accommodation. The community rehabilitation patients will need a greater input from GPs as there are often high levels of physical health problems related to lifestyle and previous poor access to primary care. Specialist Primary Care Psychiatrist posts have developed to work directly with GP practices.

Community Mental Health Team (CMHT) and outpatient psychiatry

CMHTs developed over the last 30–40 years as the large psychiatric hospitals closed. These teams were initially led by Community Psychiatric Nurses with an emphasis on patients having medication reviews (e.g. depot antipsychotic medication and Lithium Clinics), but have developed to be multidisciplinary with social workers, occupational therapists, psychologists, support workers and psychiatrists. The majority of patients are on the Care Programme Approach (CPA), which aims to have a care coordinator for those with complex mental and social health care needs. Many previously hospital-based Outpatient Clinics are now embedded within the CMHT. CPA is at the core of the operations of the CMHTs and this has recently been updated (Refocusing the Care Programme Approach, 2008), to more explicitly involve the GP, and to include social care needs, carers' needs and physical health needs.

Most referrals are sent directly to CMHTs, although in some places separate outpatient psychiatric clinics still operate. In many areas all referrals are dealt with through a 'single point of entry'. CMHT referrals are often seen by an Assessment sub-team without necessarily having an assessment from a psychiatrist, so GPs should make a purposeful request in their referral to have a consultant psychiatrist assessment if they think this is indicated.

Pathways from primary care to secondary care

The neat division between the hospital and the GP no longer exists. With the development of so many mental health teams outside of the hospital, and care being provided by Social and Health Partnerships and Third Sector organisations, there can be confusion of who to refer to. The local single point of referral or entry to community secondary mental health care has been adopted by many localities, but at the same time some groups of GP practices have developed a very close link with their local Community Mental Heath Team and continue to build on the historical and interpersonal relationships. The single point of entry can erode this successful interpersonal relationship and needs to be carefully considered before discarding for a reductionism which some reports say may have already impoverished mental health services (St John-Smith *et al.*, 2009). Continuity of care with a doctor who knows the patient's history; the doctor having an understanding of the patient; and a relationship with trusted hospital staff are rated by inpatients in importance of 1, 2 and 3 in a detailed survey of healthcare needs (Boyd, 2007).

For GPs the first point of call for known patients should usually be the CMHT, but in emergencies this should be the Crisis Team or to direct the patient and their family to the local Emergency Department, where access to psychiatric care is provided as an emergency. People who may be developing a schizophrenic disorder should be referred to EIS, as a long duration of untreated illness can lead to long-term social and health morbidity.

Case vignette: suggestions for management

- There are various services available including A&E (psychiatric emergency services) and the Crisis and Home Treatment Team. Other appropriate teams include Perinatal Psychiatry, Early Intervention and the CMHT.
- The referral can be discussed by ringing your locality psychiatrist or CMHT. Positive risk taking (being client-centred) is not appropriate, as the *child's needs are paramount*, with an urgent referral to the Child and Family Safeguarding Team and HTT (gatekeeping to inpatient care). Insight into depression or psychosis may be impaired, and the family may collude in delaying an urgent referral.
- Note the cultural barriers and language (use an advocate if available), be empathetic, respect confidentiality and religious wishes and consider stigma. The family's education and cultural integration need to be considered. Consider your own insight and professional duties. Broker a power sharing between family, patient and the requirement for safety of the patient and her daughter.

Key points

- The NICE guidelines for schizophrenia (2009) make expectations for treatment to be delivered within a community/primary care interface, with early detection and treatment with antipsychotic medication (either typical or atypical) the best evidence to decrease future morbidity and disability.
- All community mental health teams attempt to involve the family/patient in setting the care plan early. Do not assume that a cultural barrier limits your responsibility.
- In community psychiatry, treatment is increasingly being delivered with an assertive model (may involve the new Community Treatment Orders under the Mental Health Act 2007), so as to decrease social exclusion and poor access to health care.
- Maintain and develop the partnership with your CMHT, as patients value continuity of care. A single referral point of entry should not detract from knowing your locality psychiatrist and CMHT.
- Most community mental health service developments have occurred within a policy framework rather than being evidence-based, but these functional teams are set to expand for the foreseeable future, with payment by results care pathways based on diagnosis.

Further reading and bibliography

Boyd, J. (2007) *The 2006 In-Patients Importance Study*. Picker Institute Europe (http://www.nhssurveys.org.survey/486).

Department of Health (2001) *The Mental Health Policy Implementation Guide*. Department of Health, London.

Department of Health (2008) *Refocusing the Care Programme Approach: Policy and Positive Practice Guidance*. Department of Health, London.

Department of Health (1999) *National Service Framework for Mental Health: Modern Standards and Service Models*. Department of Health, London.

Stein, L. I. and Santos, A. B. (1998) *Assertive Community Treatment of Persons with Severe Mental Illness*. W. W. Norton, London and New York.

St John-Smith, P., McQueen, D., Michael, A., Ikkos, G., Maier, M. *et al.* (2009). The trouble with NHS psychiatry in England. *Psychiatric Bulletin*, **33**, 219–25.

CHAPTER 14

Risk assessment and management

Anthony Kerman and Andrew Crombie

Case history 1

Ms B is a 36-year-old single parent with a long history of periodic involvement with specialist mental health services and diagnoses of Unstable Emotional Personality Disorder and brittle insulin-dependent diabetes. She has a history since teen years of cutting her wrists when distressed and has taken three overdoses of paracetamol in the past, requiring active intervention. She lost her job as a filing clerk six months ago. She presents along with her 14-year-old son. She becomes rapidly tearful and her son confides that they are now threatened with eviction. She has self-harmed twice in the last three days; on the second occasion her son had to call an ambulance and she required sutures (which is unusual for her). She did not wait to see the psychiatric liaison team in the accident and emergency department. She says she has become increasingly despairing of life and has been having thoughts about taking a further overdose or taking all of her insulin whilst her son is at school.

Case history 2

Mr M is a 46-year-old who attends surgery with an infected wound on his right hand. He burnt himself a week earlier when he used his bare hand to lift a cup of soup he had balanced over a gas stove to heat. He smells strongly of alcohol, and admits to drinking 500 ml of vodka per day since being released from prison six months ago, having served 25 years for the manslaughter of his stepfather who had allegedly abused him. He feels low, but appetite and sleep are good and although he admits to suicidal ideation at times he denies any intent or planning. He

> has been housed in bedsit hostel accommodation and does not like living independently. He has a cousin living in the area but they are not currently speaking after an argument about money. He sees his probation officer every 2–4 weeks.

Introduction

Risk is central to all general practice but can be especially fraught in conjunction with psychiatric ill health. In part this is because, once risks have been identified, their management will not necessarily remove all risk but requires decisions regarding degrees of acceptable risk. And what is acceptable is to some extent a much broader social issue. Risks, particularly those affecting the general public or vulnerable people, have become heavily politicised and widely discussed in the media.

When beginning to think about risks it can be helpful to separate risks to the patient themselves from risks to others, and to consider explicit or latent risks. Explicit risks are raised directly by patients or others in clinical interactions (e.g. presenting requesting help with self-harm). It is important, however, also to be alert to latent risks which may not be immediately presented but are important to identify (e.g. risk of self-neglect or emotional neglect of children). We will begin by discussing approaches to assessing risk in increasing levels of detail before moving on to discuss the implications for managing both acute and chronic risks for individual clinicians and practices as a whole.

Approaches to risk assessment

Routine screening

Clearly not every consultation with a patient will necessarily raise issues of psychiatric risk. However, the issue should remain prominent in clinicians' minds. Some basic questions should be incorporated into consultations with a clear mental health focus. As a minimum patients should be asked explicitly about thoughts of self-harm. Also, where patients have made specific suggestive statements or there is a high index of suspicion, threats to others should be actively discussed.

> ## Box 14.1 Questioning about suicide risk
>
> 1. How do you see the future?
> 2. Do you feel life is worthwhile?
> 3. Have you had thoughts of harming yourself?
> 4. What have you thought of doing?
> 5. Have you made any plans to do this/how would you do this?
> 6. Is there anything preventing you from doing this?

Both lines of questioning may often be difficult to initiate, so it is often helpful to attempt to 'normalise' such feelings with a brief pre-emptive statement before embarking (e.g. 'often when patients have had a difficult time...' or 'it sounds like that person has made you really angry...'). Using a standard format of questioning can be useful (see Box 14.1).

Actuarial risk

Much effort has been devoted in recent decades to identifying, through statistical analysis, specific factors which predict an increased risk in patients for particular adverse outcomes (e.g. completed suicide, child abuse). While debate continues to rage over the relative merits of this so called 'actuarial' approach compared to so-called 'clinical judgement' alone, a familiarity with known risk factors (see Table 14.1) is undoubtedly helpful in prompting clinicians to explicitly consider risk in particular patients, both in terms of immediate risk and in identifying future potential threats.

Contextual factors

Bearing in mind actuarial factors, patients must clearly be considered within their broader circumstances. A thorough knowledge of the patient and their background is indispensable, as some understanding of a patient's life experiences, development and the quality of past interpersonal relationships will clearly inform your understanding of their likely response to current or future stressors.

General practitioners are often ideally placed to consider risks in context because of their broader knowledge of the patient's life and social circumstances. It is important to consider what means of support are available to

Table 14.1 Actuarial risk factors.

Risk of completed suicide	Risk of violence	Risk of elder abuse	Risk of child abuse
■ Male sex ■ Recent loss ■ Recent mental health inpatient discharge ■ Suicidal behaviour in 1st degree relative ■ Major depressive episode ■ Emotionally unstable personality disorder ■ Substance abuse	■ Previous history of violence ■ Rootlessness ■ Poor compliance with treatment ■ Substance misuse ■ Threat/control override symptoms ■ Specific threats made by patient ■ Access to victims	■ Sole carer ■ Carer depression ■ Carer substance abuse ■ Dementia in dependent ■ Previous history of domestic violence ■ Verbal or physical aggression from dependent ■ Shared living arrangement with carer	■ History previous abuse ■ Childhood experience of abuse in carer ■ Domestic violence ■ Substance misuse in carer ■ Children with disability ■ Children aged 0–3 years ■ Poverty/severe financial strain ■ Social isolation/ single parenting

the patient through family, friends or other professionals (or conversely where such involvement might be antagonistic). Furthermore, where the patient has formal or informal carer responsibilities these should be considered early, both as potential aggravating factors and to ensure they are specifically addressed as part of the management plan.

Inevitably risk assessment is often undertaken in the context of a specific threat or crisis. It is helpful for the patient as well as the clinician to explore the reality of the situation, the intractability of problems and the possibilities for future improvement or deterioration. Where a number of stressors exist it might also be helpful to consider their relative importance. A detailed understanding of the current stressor or threat and the patient's experience of it will be important. In these cases conducting a brief mental state examination may help give a clinician perspective on how a patient's risk may relate to their broader emotional state. Patients may well have an existing mental health condition and it is important to consider how well controlled their condition is at the time and what level of insight a patient may have into their current difficulties.

Where a psychiatric history exists, knowledge of diagnoses, previous involvement with mental health services, the quality of those interactions, previous treatments and treatment concordance should be sought and documented. A history of risk behaviour, including specific details of risk incidents (chronology, circumstances, method and mental state), is also informative.

Comorbid drug or alcohol use may often be either a causative/exacerbating factor or indeed a common coping mechanism and is important to identify. If there is a forensic history this may give some insight as to whether threatened risks have previously been acted upon. Other general medical comorbidities may pose immediate risks and will need to be considered. Conversely, it is important to remember that a patient's psychiatric ill health will often put them at greater long-term medical risk either through poor control of known conditions such as diabetes or through poorer uptake of screening opportunities and general health promotion.

A patient's religious and socio-cultural milieu will also influence their level of risk or how they might respond to particular life stressors.

Detailed questioning about specific risks

Where a specific threat or suspicion has been identified through routine questioning, a more detailed history should be taken. Where the risk is of actual intentional harm both plan and intent should be clarified. As far as the patient allows, it is important to clarify the nature and level of detail of any plan. Consideration should be given to the feasibility of the actions (i.e. opportunity and access to means such as medication or weapons). Furthermore, the clinician should explore with the patient their degree of intent to enact the plan, including their level of commitment and immediacy. Where risks are more general or unintentional (e.g. neglect) it is important to explicitly raise these concerns with the patient to explore how aware they (and those around them) are of these potential threats. Where the risk involves others (particularly children and vulnerable adults) it is often advisable to seek corroborative history from those who know the patient well to ensure the clinician is fully informed of all the factors.

Risk assessment tools

A number of formal risk assessment tools have been developed and the variety available can seem overwhelming. Formal tools may be for specific types of risk (e.g. forensic, child abuse). They are now routinely used in specialist mental health services but vary considerably in their length and level of detail. Thus when selecting an appropriate risk assessment tool both predictive values and ease of use (particularly in a primary care setting) should be considered. Given the inherent time pressures they may be of limited value in general practice but could be of use for patients with high and complex risk.

Managing risk

There will be many situations in which risk management will actually be crisis management as a patient presents with a new problem or unexpected deterioration. We will begin by considering these before moving on to longer term risks.

Initial approach to the patient

Personal safety should be implicit in your approach to the patient. You should ensure your environment is safe and remain alert to early indicators of violence developing in the consultation. The immediate approach to the patient will rely on excellent communication skills. A range of components of good communication, such as an open style and active listening can be used to show sympathy and empathy and in doing so may help to diffuse a situation. In conjunction with a careful, thorough assessment it may be possible to reframe problems in such a way as to reduce anxiety and escalation of risk.

It may be that early pharmacological intervention is required and benzodiazepines are commonly used in the short term while antipsychotic medication may be more appropriate in certain circumstances. Conversely, removal of medication or limitation of its availability may be needed if it has been implicated in a planned overdose attempt. Similarly, other means of planned harm to self or others may need to be attended to.

Making use of local resources

Inherent in general practice is a limit on the time that can be spent in a single appointment and consequently there is a role as gatekeeper both for further appointments at the practice and for onward referral. It is important to be aware of these limitations and remember that it is appropriate to refer on for further assessment.

It may be that the patient needs to be removed from their current situation. Although in some situations this may be possible by engaging a supportive family or social network, more often it will involve shared care with referral to the psychiatric team. Options will include both admission to a psychiatric ward (voluntary or compulsory) as well as urgent assessment and treatment via the crisis team or single-point-of-access service (depending on local arrangements) to facilitate alternatives to admission. In less urgent cases, routine referral to the local CMHT or intake/assessment team may be more appropriate. There are also local variations with some areas having access to residential respite facilities. In situations involving threatened violence to others or levels of aggression that cannot be managed or talked down it may be necessary to involve the police. A further break in patient confidentiality may be required to inform the target subject of any specific threats.

There are many other resources available in the community including drug and alcohol support teams and voluntary sector organisations providing key work, counselling, activities and training. Local pharmacies and controlled prescribing guidelines can be involved to limit a patient's access to medications.

Remember to consider social support for the patient but also for any dependants such as children who may live with the patient or elderly relatives who may rely on the patient for some level of support. This may require involving local social services and in critical cases will be mandatory.

Longer term risks

Many risks identified will be chronic or potential future risks. Thinking of the longer term it is important to think broadly about the whole person and their social context. Management will involve working with patients on identifying strategies to lessen their risk. It may take the form of education and psychological support, such as anxiety or anger management courses, longer-term psychological interventions or key working. Support can be organised on a one-to-one basis or as group work. It is therefore important to familiarise oneself with local statutory and voluntary organisations providing services for mental health.

There may be a need for ongoing pharmacological treatment with allowances made for levels of concordance (e.g. oral medications versus injections).

Social support is a common thread in risk management plans, as very often precipitants for threatened risk are issues such as financial difficulties or housing problems. Awareness of potential precipitants and timely intervention may help avert a crisis. This might involve supporting patients to access local social services or voluntary sector advice (e.g. Citizen's Advice Bureau).

Where patients are under the care of specialist mental health services, much of the longer-term planning role may be fulfilled by the mental health team. The patient will be subject to a Care Programme Approach (CPA) where their care needs are regularly assessed and plans made to address them (for patients seen solely in outpatient clinics this may take the form of a plan documented in the clinic letter). GP communication with this process will involve invitations to attend CPA meetings or contribute information in writing. It is important to remain alert to any gaps in care which may require communication with the team and to ensure that care plans are noted in the patient's record.

Statutory risk management structures

Mandatory reporting arrangements in cases involving serious risks to children are in place in the UK. Structures also exist for reporting concerns regarding vulnerable adults and for managing patients who are considered to be at high risk of offending. It is important to be aware of these statutory arrangements and to remain up to date with any changes (see Table 14.2).

Issues for the GP and practice

A multitude of issues have been discussed, focusing on the patient's risks and their management, but a GP must also consider broader practice issues such as the need to provide themselves and staff with a safe working environment equipped with easy to use emergency alarms and physically arranged to allow escape if necessary. Trained staff should be available to act as chaperones.

Where possible the practice should endeavour to facilitate continuity of care, which will be affected by appointment systems as well as the balance of partners and regular salaried GPs verses locum staff. When this is not possible the computerised medical record allows for information to be shared while also enabling ready use of patient registers and the Quality and Outcomes Frame-

Table 14.2 Statutory arrangement for risk management (England and Wales).

Statutory arrangement	Comments
Safeguarding Children	Formal arrangements for protecting children at risk of abuse or neglect. Coordinated by Local Authority social services. Mandatory reporting for suspected abuse or neglect
Safeguarding of Vulnerable Adults (SOVA)	Arrangements for preventing abuse and neglect of vulnerable adults (e.g. mentally ill, vulnerable elderly people, people with learning disabilities). Coordinated by Local Authority. No mandatory reporting. Reporting based on 'best interest' principles and assessments of capacity to consent ('Caldicott principles')
Multi-Agency Public Protection Arrangements (MAPPA)	Arrangements for coordinated assessment and risk management of the most serious sexual and violent offenders in the community. Involve multiple sectors (police, probation, social services, health). Information-sharing, monitoring and minimising risk (e.g. through social support) are key components.

work to facilitate health promotion. The appointment system should allow sufficient time for proper assessment. Issues such as these should be actively managed, but meetings should also allow sufficient flexibility to raise any concerns as they arise. There should also be a practice policy for significant event analysis, including reviews of any changes made as a result of them.

Individual GPs have responsibility for doctor specific issues such as maintaining a suitable set of skills and up-to-date knowledge to be able to safely assess and manage risk. The doctor also has a legal responsibility to record full and contemporaneous records. As well as their role in patient care these will be required if there are any doubts about care or even the prospect of litigation. Medical indemnity is an absolute requirement.

Conclusion

The basis of risk assessment is a return to the first principles of a full history and mental state examination. This allows specific questioning about risk and detection of risk factors or red flags in the context of the patient's past and present life experiences.

Good communication is the cornerstone of risk management both with the patient and the wider mental health, social services and voluntary sectors. This process is facilitated by expecting risks to present and being prepared with appropriate working practice systems and knowledge of locally available resources.

Key points

- When presented with a patient at risk, remember that a full assessment of risk will require assimilation of multiple physical, psychological and social factors. Be thorough.
- There may be only yourself and the patient in the consulting room, but remember you do not need to make decisions in isolation. Make use of the multidisciplinary team, referring if necessary and maintaining good communication.
- Have a clear plan managing both a crisis and longer-term risks including strategies for the unexpected ('safety net' with emergency numbers for important contacts).
- Ensure there is planned follow up and that you know when, how and by whom.
- Document all interactions and decisions thoroughly.

Further reading and bibliography

Department of Health and Home Office (2000) *No Secrets: Guidance on Developing and Implementing Policies and Procedures to Protect Vulnerable Adults From Abuse*. Department of Health, London.

Gaynes, B. *et al.* (2004) Screening for suicide risk in adults: a summary of the evidence for the U.S. Preventative Services Task Force. *Annals of Internal Medicine*, **140**, 822–35.

HM Government (2007) *Statutory Guidance on Making Arrangements to Safeguard and Promote the Welfare of Children Under Section 11 of the Children Act 2004*. Department for Education and Skills, London.

Holloway, R. (2004) Risk: more questions than answers. *Advances in Psychiatric Treatment*, **10**, 273–4.

Home Office (2003) *MAPPA Guidance*. Home Office, London.

Legislation

CHAPTER 15

Consent and capacity

Diana Andrea Barron and Adrian Raby

> ## Case history 1
>
> Peter is 68 years old. He has bipolar affective disorder. He recently recovered from an episode of severe depression and attends your surgery requesting a 'health MOT'. During the consultation you note that he appears elated and ask him about his mood, sleep, appetite and energy levels. It emerges that Peter feels '110%'. He tells you his energy levels are so good that he only needs 4 hours sleep a night. He is surprised that he has gained 15 kilos since his last visit to your surgery and attributes this to his partner's extraordinarily good cooking.
>
> You explain to Peter that you think he seems elated and ask him if he would be happy to change his current medication and attend your surgery in a week's time. Peter agrees stating he would do anything to avoid another admission to 'that dreadful hospital'.
>
> You initiate a reducing regimen of his dose of Selective Serotonin Reuptake Inhibitor (SSRI) and arrange appropriate follow-up.
>
> ## Case history 2
>
> Gina has bipolar affective disorder. She is 25 years old and has been well for two years. She would like to start a family with her husband, to whom she has been married for the past 18 months. She and her mother-in-law have come to your surgery to ask for prenatal advice. She is currently taking sodium valproate as a mood stabiliser; she would like to stop this medication. Her mother-in-law is also keen for this to be stopped.
>
> You talk to Gina about her general health, her current medication and the risks of continuing her current medication in addition to the

risks of discontinuing them. You provide her with written information and arrange a further appointment for her to meet you to discuss matters on her own.

Case history 3

Mark is 55, he has Down's Syndrome and moderate learning disability. He has no known relatives and has lived in residential care all his life. His carers have reported that there has been a deterioration in his self-care skills over the past year. He has been reviewed by the community consultant psychiatrist for people with learning disability, who has diagnosed probable Alzheimer's dementia and has advised you to request an MRI of his brain and to start a cholinesterase inhibitor. Mark's carers tell you that Mark will not go into the MRI suite; Mark has previously required a general anaesthetic in order to undergo dental work.

You meet with Mark and find that he lacks mental capacity to consent to a general anaesthetic or to start a new medication. You refer Mark to the IMCA (Independent Mental Capacity Advocate) service and convene a meeting with all Mark's carers, the IMCA, the community psychiatrist and others involved in Mark's care and those who know Mark well in order to decide what would be in Mark's best interests.

Introduction

This chapter aims to provide GPs with information about capacity and consent as they relate to mental health issues in the primary care setting. The chapter focuses solely on adults within England and Wales.

Informed consent is a common law defence against battery: the touching of a person without his or her consent. For example giving an individual a general anaesthetic without the patient's consent could constitute battery. If the physician can show that the individual had given valid consent this would be a defence against any such claim.

The process of gaining valid consent is a cornerstone of good medical practice and represents the means by which patients are able to make autonomous decisions. Valid consent to treatment requires that consent be given voluntarily by an appropriately informed person who has capacity to consent to the intervention/treatment in question. This process is summarised in Figure 15.1.

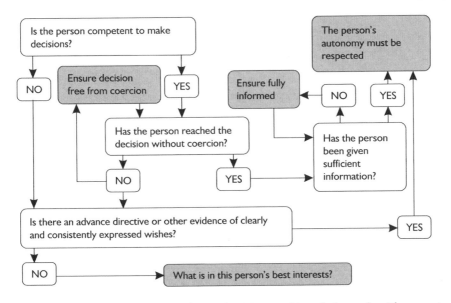

Figure 15.1 Decision-making about decision-making (adapted with permission from Professor Tom Sensky).

In the context of mental health these guiding principles remain the same. However, legislation can render mental health care decision making a special case, specifically in relation to:

- Medication
- Admission to hospital
- Treatment in the community

The amended Mental Health Act 1983 (MHA) sets out the circumstances in which a person may be detained or treated for a mental disorder without their consent and is discussed in detail in Chapter 16.

Voluntariness

Consent must be freely given. To be legally valid there must not be undue external pressures or coercion. Coercion can normally be distinguished from appropriate reassurance or advice about treatment (Department of Health, 2009). Additional sources of coercion specific to mental health include the perceived threat of involuntary admission to hospital under the auspices of the MHA. In Case study 1, Peter refers to 'that dreadful hospital'. It is not clear from the facts whether Peter considers that he is being threatened with admission and if his decision to accept the changes to his medication regimen would have been different had he not thought he was going to be admitted. It is the clinician's responsibility to clarify this point. Assuming that a patient such as Peter has capacity to make decisions, and does not fulfil the criteria for treatment under the Mental Health Act, his GP has a duty to ensure that his decisions are made freely; otherwise any consent in such circumstances may not be valid.

Sources of coercion can also come from carers, friends or family. GPs should be alert to this possibility and where appropriate should arrange to see the person on their own in order to establish that the decision is truly the patient's own, as in Case 2.

Some individuals can be easily influenced and are therefore likely to give the response to questions that they believe is expected of them. While this does not necessarily indicate coercion it might imply that there is an impairment of the individual's ability to use information given in order to make a decision. Again clinicians should be aware of this possibility. An example of this could occur in the context of a person with a mild learning disability.

Appropriately informed

To give valid consent an individual should have received sufficient information about the nature and purpose of the intervention. Whilst this degree of information is sufficient to defend a charge of battery, in healthcare decision making clinicians have a wider professional duty to provide additional information about the range of treatment options, their relative risks, burdens and likelihood of success in order to ensure that patients are genuinely informed. Moreover, should a risk or side-effect of treatment materialise of which the patient was not made aware the doctor may be open to a claim of negligence. Clinicians can access guidelines about what information should be given to patients when helping them to make any clinical decision. The basic requirements are set out in guidance from the General Medical Council (GMC, 2009) and the British Medical Association (BMA, 2009).

The guidance emphasises that all medical decisions should be made in partnership with patients. Therefore clinicians must:

- Listen to patients and respect the patient's own views about their health
- Discuss with patients what their diagnosis, prognosis, treatment and care involve

- Share with patients the information they want or need in order to make decisions
- Maximise patients' opportunities, and their ability, to make decisions for themselves
- Respect patients' decisions

The amount of information and detail required varies according to the individual circumstances and the decision in hand. Topics that should be covered are summarised in Box 15.1.

In Case 2 the clinician has informed Gina of the risks of continuing her current medications which would include the risk of teratogenicity (cardio-

---

Box 15.1 GMC guidance on information for patients

As a clinician you should consider discussing:

(a) the diagnosis and prognosis

(b) any uncertainties about the diagnosis or prognosis, including options for further investigations

(c) options for treating or managing the condition, including the option not to treat

(d) the purpose of any proposed investigation or treatment and what it will involve

(e) the potential benefits, risks and burdens, and the likelihood of success, for each option; this should include information, if available, about whether the benefits or risks are affected by which organisation or doctor is chosen to provide care

(f) whether a proposed investigation or treatment is part of a research programme or is an innovative treatment designed specifically for their benefit

(g) the people who will be mainly responsible for and involved in their care, what their roles are, and to what extent students may be involved

(h) their right to refuse to take part in teaching or research

(i) their right to seek a second opinion

(j) any bills they will have to pay

(k) any conflicts of interest that you, or your organisation, may have

(l) any treatments that you believe have greater potential benefit for the patient than those you or your organisation can offer

---

vascular malformations and neural tube defects), in addition to the risks of discontinuing them (i.e. the potential risks associated with a relapse of her bipolar disorder). Alternative courses of action should also be discussed, such as reducing the dose of sodium valproate used or the introduction of an antipsychotic medication as an alternative mood stabiliser. (Refer to NICE guidance (2006), and Chapter 8 for further detail.)

Where an individual is unable to make a decision, for example if they lack mental capacity, or are subject to statutory provision, for example under the Mental Health Act, it is also good practice to provide information and to involve them in the decision-making process as far as is possible.

Information must be given in a format that can be understood by the patient. This may require an interpreter in the case of those who do not speak English or a British Sign Language Interpreter for those with hearing impairments. Where an individual has impaired comprehension due to a learning disability or neurological disorder, information must be provided in an easily understandable format. The Mental Capacity Act Code of Practice states that to help someone make a decision for themselves, all possible and appropriate means of communication should be tried (Department of Constitutional Affairs, 2007). Furthermore, the patient should be supported to communicate their questions and decision as far as possible. This most commonly will be through verbal means, although sign language and gestures may be sufficient.

Mental capacity

Where an individual lacks mental capacity to make a decision they are unable to give valid consent. The definition of mental capacity, its assessment and the process for decision-making on behalf of an individual lacking mental capacity are set out in the Mental Capacity Act (2005). The Act, which came into force in 2007, is an extremely important piece of legislation both in guiding medical decision makers and in potentially shaping the doctor–patient relationship where the patient lacks full capacity. The Act codifies the pre-existing case law and other sources of good practice that relate to the management of decision making for people who lack capacity, and includes guiding principles (Box 15.2).

Everyone is presumed to have capacity unless they are unable to make a decision because of a disturbance or impairment of functioning of the mind (Box 15.3). However nobody should be labelled 'incapable' as a result of having a particular medical condition or diagnosis. There is no single attribute, such as a person's age, appearance or any particular behavioural condition or aspect of their behaviour, that can establish lack of capacity.

Box 15.2 Guiding principles for interpretation and application of the Mental Capacity Act

1. Presumption of capacity
All adults have a right to make their own decisions and must be assumed to have capacity unless it is proven otherwise.

2. Help people to make decision themselves
There is a general right for individuals to be supported to make their own decisions, i.e. people must be given all appropriate help before it is concluded they cannot make their own decisions.

3. Unwise decisions may be OK
Individuals retain the right to make what seem to be eccentric or unwise decisions.

4. Best interests are always paramount
Anything done for or on behalf of people who lack capacity must be in their best interests

5. Least restrictive action
Anything done for or on behalf of people who lack capacity should be the least restrictive on their basic rights and freedoms.

Box 15.3 Examples of disturbance or impairment of the mind

- Conditions associated with some forms of mental illness
- Dementia
- Significant learning disabilities
- The long-term effects of brain damage
- Physical or medical conditions that cause confusion
- Drowsiness or loss of consciousness
- Delirium
- Concussion following a head injury
- The symptoms of alcohol or drug use

An individual has capacity if they can understand the information relevant to that decision, and retain that information, and use or weigh up that information, and communicate their decision. If any of these elements are absent then the person is deemed to lack capacity:

1. Understand the information relevant to that decision

This can only be assessed after the relevant information has been given to the individual. Time and effort must be made to ensure that the information is appropriate and accessible according to the individual's abilities and level of understanding. Options to assess an individual's understanding include asking the individual if they have any questions about the intervention or asking the individual to explain what they understand about the intervention being offered. For example, in Case 1 the GP will have explained to Peter that there is a need to stop SSRIs and the rationale for using a reducing regimen to avoid any discontinuation symptoms. The GP could ask Peter about his understanding of the features of any discontinuation symptoms and encourage a general discussion about the risks of stopping SSRIs.

2. Retain that information

The individual needs to hold the information in their mind long enough for them to be able to make the decision in hand.

3. Use or weigh up the information

An individual may be able to understand the information but be unable to use the information in the process of decision making. An example of this is severe depression, where an individual's cognitive distortions can cause their thinking to be so clouded by negative thoughts that they may not be able to come to a decision about treatment.

4. Communicate their decision

An individual must be able to communicate their decision to the clinician. However, before deciding that an individual is unable to communicate it is essential to show that all practical steps to maximise an individual's ability to do so have been taken. This may require referral to secondary services for input from speech and language therapy, clinical psychology or other disciplines if the appropriate expertise is available. Where an individual is unable to communicate their decision in any way at all they are deemed to lack mental capacity.

Capacity is regarded as 'decision specific', i.e. someone may lack capacity to take a decision about one aspect of their life but are capable of deciding about another, or they may be capable of it at one point in time but not at another time. An example of the former is given in Case 3. Mark is an individual with a moderate learning disability; therefore he may have the mental capacity to choose to join in an activity but not have the mental capacity to decide whether to start a new medication. An example of a situation where a person's capacity may fluctuate would be an acute confusional state. If a person is likely to regain capacity and it is safe to defer the decision to a later point in time then the decision should normally be deferred.

Management of those lacking capacity

Where an individual lacks the mental capacity to make a decision for themselves, the Mental Capacity Act governs the circumstances in which a decision can be made on their behalf. (See also Box 15.4 on Lasting Power of Attorney and Box 15.5 on Advance directives.)

Box 15.4 Lasting Power of Attorney

Lasting Powers of Attorney are a way for an individual to delegate decision-making powers to another person. In general they are the principal means for an individual to choose who will manage their affairs, and under what conditions. There are two types of Power of Attorney, one relating to property/financial matters and the other relating to the welfare of the individual including medical matters. The Mental Capacity Act sets out how to create and administer a Lasting Power of Attorney and its registration.

Box 15.5 Advance directives

The Mental Capacity Act also governs the use of advance directives which are made by people when they have capacity in relation to decisions when they may lack capacity in the future. Section 26(1) provides that if an individual has made an advance decision which is both valid and applicable to the treatment in question after the individual loses capacity, then the directive has the same force as if the decision maker has capacity. Certain types of decision have additional requirements. The decision to decline life-sustaining treatment must be in writing, signed by the individual or another person in their presence, and the signature witnessed. The decision must include the statement to the effect that it is to apply to that treatment even if life is at risk.

The responsibility for decision making rests with the person who is responsible for carrying out the procedure or treatment in question. This could be a relative, healthcare worker or social care worker. For example in Case 3 Mark's carer made the decision to bring Mark to the GP surgery.

However, where a decision relates to a serious medical intervention or change of accommodation and the individual has no close family or friends, the individual must be referred to an Independent Mental Capacity Advocate Service to appoint an Independent Mental Capacity Advocate (IMCA). Where an IMCA has been appointed, the decision maker must consider their opinion when deciding how to act in an individual's best interests.

Mental Capacity Act framework for best interests decisions

Best interests decisions are made on behalf of people who lack mental capacity to make a decision for themselves and who do not have a valid advance directive. In these instances the decision maker must make a decision that is in the person's best interests. An everyday example of a clinical decision would be the decision to start antibiotics for a urinary tract infection. In this case the decision maker is the clinician and they must determine what is in the person's best interests. The Mental Capacity Act and its Code of Practice provide clinicians with a framework to follow when doing this. This process is summarised in Figure 15.2.

When to refer to specialist services

The Mental Capacity Act provides clinicians with the tools necessary to assess mental capacity where this is indicated. In some cases it is necessary to refer to specialist services to help individuals understand the information that is given to them and/or facilitate their own ability to communicate questions and their decision to the clinician. Appropriate secondary services may include speech and language therapy or a clinical psychologist and may involve the use of accessible format materials and total communication approaches. For complex cases, psychiatrists and psychologists can provide specialist advice on the assessment of capacity – for example if a case needs to go to the Court of Protection (Box 15.6).

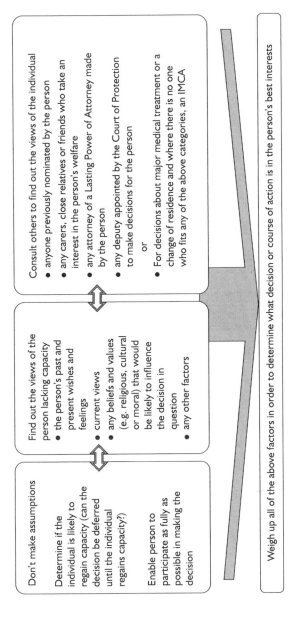

Figure 15.2 Best interests decisions.

Box 15.6 Examples of cases that need to go to the Court of Protection

- Financial decisions for a person who lacks capacity to make that decision and who has no EPA/LPA in place to make such a decision
- Making or altering a will on behalf of a person who lacks capacity to do so
- Where there is genuine doubt or disagreement about the existence, validity or applicability of an advance decision to refuse treatment
- Where there is a major disagreement regarding a serious decision (e.g. declining life-prolonging treatment)
- Where a family carer or a solicitor asks for personal information about someone who lacks capacity to consent to that information being given
- Where someone suspects that a person who lacks capacity to make decisions to protect themselves is at risk of harm or abuse from a named individual.

Key points

- The process of gaining valid consent is a cornerstone of good medical practice and represents the means by which patients are able to make autonomous decisions.
- Clinicians need to be aware of circumstances where pressure may be brought to bear on patients, and must take steps to minimise the risk of coercion in the decision-making process.
- The Mental Capacity Act provides clinicians with the tools necessary to assess mental capacity and to treat those who lack capacity.
- It is essential to provide information to and involve in the decision-making process, individuals who lack mental capacity or who are treated under the Mental Health Act.
- Time and effort must be made to ensure that the communication of information is appropriate and accessible according to the individual's abilities and level of understanding which may involve referral to specialist services.

Further reading and bibliography

British Medical Association Consent Tool Kit (2009) BMA, London. http://www. bma.org.uk/images/consenttoolkitdec2009_tcm41-193139.pdf. Accessed 16 July 2010.

Department of Health (2009) *Reference Guide to Consent for Examination or Treatment*, 2nd edn. Department of Health, London. http://www.dh.gov.uk/en/Publicationsandstatistics/Publications/PublicationsPolicyAndGuidance/DH_103643. Accessed 16 July 2010.

Department for Constitutional Affairs (2007) *Mental Capacity Act Code of Practice*. Stationery Office, London. http://www.dca.gov.uk/legal-policy/mental-capacity/mca-cp.pdf. Accessed 16 July 2010.

General Medical Council (2009) *Consent: Patients and Doctors Making Decisions Together*. GMC: London. http://www.gmc-uk.org/guidance/ethical_guidance/consent_guidance_index.asp. Accessed 16 July 2010.

NICE (2006) *The Management of Bipolar Disorder in Adults, Children and Adolescents, in Primary and Secondary Care*. Clinical guidelines CG38. National Institute of Clinical and Health Excellence. http://guidance.nice.org.uk/CG38.

Thank you to Professor Tom Sensky (Consultant Psychiatrist, Imperial College London) for providing permission to adapt Figure 15.1.

CHAPTER 16

Using the Mental Health Act

Afia Ali, Ian Hall and Andrew Dicker

Case history

The partner of a 48-year-old gentleman makes an urgent call to his GP. She is concerned about his behaviour and her own welfare. He has become increasingly jealous and has been accusing her of having an affair with her boss. He routinely searches her belongings for evidence of the affair and today has been making threats of harming her after finding a shirt button in her purse, which he believes provides evidence of the affair. She has noticed that he has been drinking excessive amounts of alcohol and has been increasingly neglecting himself.

This is his first psychiatric presentation. His GP knows him well and contacts the duty Approved Mental Health Practitioner and arranges an urgent mental health act assessment. The GP makes the second medical recommendation and the patient is detained in hospital under section 2 of the Mental Health Act.

Introduction

The purpose of mental health law is to balance the need to detain people compulsorily, in order to protect them or other people from harm, and the need to respect people's right to self-determination. The new Mental Health Act 2007, which applies to England and Wales, substantially amends the Mental Health Act 1983. Amendments include changes to the definition of mental disorder, changes to the roles of professionals and the introduction of supervised community treatment. A new Code of Practice is now available and provides guidance on how these changes should be applied in clinical practice. Fortunately, most of these changes do not affect GPs directly, as the process of making medical recommendations has not changed. However, GPs should be familiar with some of the more important changes in order to ensure that appropriate care is provided, in particular for patients receiving care in the community.

The role of GPs

Mental health problems such as depression and anxiety are common in the community and GPs have a significant role in providing care for patients with mental health needs. GPs are regularly asked to both arrange and undertake mental health act assessments for possible compulsory detention in hospital for assessment (section 2) or treatment (section 3). The role of the GP during assessments is important as they may be the only person to have previously known the patient. GPs are likely to have detailed knowledge of the patient's medical history and personal circumstances, which are relevant to making a decision about whether compulsory detention may be in the best interests of the patient and what other options should be explored.

Conducting a Mental Health Act assessment

Initiating a Mental Health Act assessment

GPs may be approached by a concerned relative, a carer or a member of the community mental health team about a person with mental health needs. A review of the patient should be arranged in the first instance and, if appropriate, a review by a consultant psychiatrist should be requested. If a mental health act assessment is required, this can be arranged following the consultant review. If there are concerns about the safety of the patient (e.g. self-neglect or suicide risk) or about the safety of others (e.g. physical aggression, sexual exploitation), and the patient is refusing to consent to an informal admission to hospital, an urgent mental health act assessment may need to be arranged by the GP. The duty Approved Mental Health Practitioner (AMHP), formerly known as the Approved Social Worker (ASW) will need to be contacted and the case will then be discussed to determine whether a Mental Health Act assessment is warranted. The AMHP may then request the GP to carry out a medical examination, if appropriate, including a mental state examination, and if appropriate, provide a written medical recommendation for compulsory detention of the patient under the terms of the Act.

Making medical recommendations

There are detailed guidelines about GPs making medical recommendations published by the Department of Health (2001). This is a good reference source, particularly for GPs who have had little experience in carrying out assessments. Most assessment and treatment sections under the mental health act require two medical recommendations (with the exception of emergency orders under section 4, where only one recommendation is required). The AMHP coordinates the assessment process, is required to interview the patient and arrive at an independent decision, irrespective of the medical recommendations, as to whether or not the patient should be detained under the Act. If the patient is to be detained for treatment (section 3) then the AMHP must consult the nearest relative as part of the decision-making process. If the patient is to be detained for assessment (section 2) then there is a duty to inform the nearest relative. If the AMHP is satisfied that compulsory detention in hospital is warranted, an application is then made to the managers of the hospital where detention will take place. Applications for compulsion can also be made by the nearest relative, although this is uncommon.

Medical recommendations are made by two doctors (registered medical practitioners) who have both examined the patient, either jointly, which is considered to be good practice, or separately. The medical examinations must be completed within five clear days of each other. The first recommendation is usually provided by a medical practitioner approved under section 12 (2) of the act, which requires that he or she has special experience in the diagnosis and treatment of mental disorders. It is good practice for the second recommendation to be made by a medical practitioner who has had 'previous acquaintance' with the patient, unless the patient is known by the first practitioner. GPs are often in a good position to undertake this role due to their prior knowledge of the patient, particularly where the patient is not known to the mental health services. It is therefore good practice, and in the best interests of the patient, for the GP to make the second recommendation. However, it is sometimes not practicable for GPs to make the second recommendation, particularly for out of hours assessments. In such circumstances the second recommendation is usually made by another section 12(2) approved doctor. It is good practice for a joint assessment to be conducted with the AMHP. GPs are entitled to claim fees for travel and for carrying out an assessment, even if a recommendation is not made.

Common sections of the 1983 Mental Health Act and amendments introduced by 2007 Act

New definition of mental disorder

One of the significant amendments to the 1983 Act is the new definition of 'mental disorder', which is now defined as 'any disorder or disability of the mind'. Although this simplifies the definition and reduces confusion over eligibility, it also increases the number of disorders that are now included within the act. Controversially, people with personality disorders, autism and disorders secondary to psycho-substance abuse (with the exception of alcohol and drug dependence), who were previously excluded, can now be compulsorily detained. However, the Act does continue to exclude people with learning disability from being detained on a treatment order unless it is associated with 'abnormally aggressive' or 'seriously irresponsible' behaviour.

Criteria for compulsion

Wherever possible, attempts should be made to admit the person informally. If patients refuse to consent to hospital admission, or are unable to consent, then compulsory admission can be considered. This requires that:

1. The person is suffering from a mental disorder that is eligible under the Act
2. The mental disorder is of a nature or degree to warrant further assessment (section 2) or medical treatment (section 3) in hospital
3. The patient needs to detained under the Act in the interest of his or her health or safety or for the protection of others

Section 2

This provides for compulsory admission for assessment in hospital (see Table 16.1). The section requires two medical recommendations and lasts up to 28 days. This section is appropriate for patients presenting for the first time with a psychiatric illness where the diagnosis remains uncertain or for those with a previous psychiatric history where the current presentation is different from previous episodes. The patient can be subsequently detained under section 3 (see below) or the patient may remain in hospital informally or be discharged.

Table 16.1 Common sections of the Mental Health Act 1983.

Section	Duration	Application process	Conditions of admission	Right of appeal	Renewal
Section 2 (admission for assessment)	Up to 28 days	Two medical recommendations. Application made by AMHP or 'nearest relative'	The person suffers from a mental disorder that is of a nature or degree to warrant assessment in hospital and the patient needs to be detained in the interest of his or her health or safety or for protection of others	Yes, within first 14 days of detention	No
Section 4 (emergency admission)	72 hours	One medical recommendation. Application by 'nearest relative' or AMHP	Urgent necessity that person is admitted and detained. Waiting for second recommendation could cause 'undesirable delay'	No	No
Section 3 (admission for treatment)	Up to 6 months	As Section 2	The person suffers from a mental disorder that is of a nature or degree to warrant treatment in hospital and the patient needs to be detained in the interest of his or her health or safety or for protection of others; 'appropriate treatment' must be available, and treatment can only be provided if the patient is admitted under section	Yes, in the first 6 months of detention. Automatic tribunal after 6 months if no appeal, then every 3 years.	Yes, 6 months and then annually
Guardianship	Up to 6 months	Two medical recommendations. Application made to local social services authority	Person suffers from a mental disorder and must be in the interest of the welfare of the patient or for the protection of others	Yes, once in first 6 months, once in second 6 months and once every year after that	Yes, 6 months and then annually

Section 3

This section enables a person with a known mental disorder to be detained for the purpose of receiving treatment. Two medical recommendations are required. An additional condition is that treatment can only be provided if the patient is detained under section 3. A patient may be detained for up to 6 months, although after 3 months the patient must give his or her consent for the treatment to continue, or must be assessed by a second opinion doctor. The section can be renewed after 6 months and again after 12 months.

One of the changes introduced by the 2007 Mental Health Act is the introduction of the 'appropriate medical treatment' test, which replaces the previous 'treatability' test. This applies to treatment sections and requires that a person is not detained unless appropriate medical treatment is available for his or her mental disorder in the specified hospital where detention is to take place. 'Medical treatment' is loosely defined and covers a range of treatments, including psychological therapy, nursing and rehabilitation, and must take into account the nature and degree of the mental disorder and the patient's circumstances. Such medical treatment must have the purpose of alleviating or preventing worsening of the mental disorder or one of its symptoms or manifestations. Previously it was a requirement that the likely effect of treatment would be to alleviate or prevent a deterioration in the mental disorder. Although this appears to be a subtle change, it is now possible for almost any disorder to be treated under the Act.

Section 4

This is an emergency section enabling a person to be detained in hospital for assessment for up to three days. It requires one medical recommendation only, which can be provided by GPs. This section is usually applied when a person needs urgent admission and it has not been possible to obtain two medical recommendations. This can then be converted later to a section 2 if appropriate.

Section 136

This section permits a police officer to bring a person who appears to be suffering from a mental disorder in a public place to a place of safety, in order for a mental health act assessment to take place. Places of safety are usually the Accident and Emergency Department, the police station, or increasingly a purpose-built section 136 suite at a psychiatric hospital. The section lasts up to

72 hours. Under the new Act, it is now possible to transfer people from places of safety to ensure that people receive appropriate care and treatment.

Section 135

This permits the police to enter a place of residence in order to remove a person suspected of having a mental disorder, to a place of safety for a mental health act assessment. An AMHP must apply to the Magistrates court for a warrant to enable the police to enter the premises. The section lasts for up to 72 hours.

Section 37/41

Section 37 is a hospital order permitting an offender convicted by the court to be admitted to hospital for treatment. Section 41 can be added to it. This is a restriction order that restricts the discharge of the patient and is for more serious or dangerous offenders. Discharge from section 41 requires the authorisation of the Secretary of State for Justice or a mental health Tribunal.

Patients already in hospitals

GPs may be asked to examine and make a second medical recommendation for a patient who was admitted informally or for a patient who was admitted under an emergency section (section 4).

Community treatment provisions

Supervised community treatment

Another significant change is the introduction of supervised community treatment. The aim is to promote treatment within the community for patients who no longer need to be in hospital to receive treatment. Patients can only be discharged with a community treatment order if they are on a treatment order (section 3, section 37 (unrestricted)). An application is made by the responsible clinician with the agreement of an AMHP. However, the patient cannot be forced to take medication in the community but may be recalled back to hospital if he or she requires treatment for their mental disorder in hospital and there is a risk to the health or safety of the patient or to others. Supervised community treatment could potentially increase the workload of GPs who may have to take a more active role in looking after the mental health needs of patients who were previously detained in hospital.

Guardianship

The purpose of a guardianship order is to ensure that a person's welfare is protected rather than to receive medical treatment. The patient must be suffering from a 'mental disorder' and it must be 'in the interests of the welfare of the patient or for the protection of other persons'. Two medical recommendations are required. The guardian is usually the local social services authority and has the power to specify where the person should live (e.g. to discourage him or her from sleeping rough), can specify that the person attends appointments with professionals at specified places and times (e.g. medical, education or training) and can require that professionals have access to the person at the place of residence.

Other changes to the Mental Health Act

Table 16.2 summarises the main amendments to the 1983 Act. One of the changes introduced into the code of practice is the introduction of five key principles, which include promoting a greater awareness of culture and diversity ('respect') and encouraging patient participation in treatment decisions ('participation and effectiveness'). There are also changes to professional roles, based on professionals achieving agreed competencies. The new AMHP, which replaces ASW, is now open to psychologists, occupational therapists and nurses as well as social workers. The role of 'responsible medical officer' has now been replaced with 'responsible clinician' and is also open to the above professionals as well as registered medical practitioners. However, a substantial amount of training will be required to achieve the required competencies and therefore only senior level professionals are likely to be able to take on this role.

A number of new safeguards for patients have been introduced, which should improve the experience of being detained under the Act. These include the right for all patients to have access to independent mental health advocates, the inclusion of civil partners as 'nearest relative' and the right for patients to displace their nearest relative.

Table 16.2 Amendments introduced by Mental Health Act 2007.

Amendment	Before 2007 amendments	After 2007 amendments
Principles	None	Five principles in Code of Practice: purpose; least restriction; respect; participation and effectiveness, efficiency and equity
Definition of mental disorder for treatment orders	Mental illness; psychopathic disorder; mental impairment and severe mental impairment	Any disorder or disability of mind
Treatment test	Likely **effects** of treatment to alleviate or prevent a deterioration in condition	**Purpose** of treatment is to alleviate or prevent a deterioration in the condition, **or one of its symptoms or manifestations** Treatment must be **available**
Person applying for orders	Approved Social Worker	Approved Mental Health Professional (nurse, social worker, psychologist, occupational therapist)
Person with overall responsibility for treatment of detained patient	Responsible Medical Officer	Responsible Clinician (must be an Approved Clinician – medical practitioner, psychologist, nurse, occupational therapist, social worker)
Compulsion for community patients	Guardianship Section 17 leave Supervised discharge	Guardianship Section 17 leave (not generally for more than a week or so) Supervised Community Treatment
Forcible administration of medication in the community	No	No
Transfers between place of safety under s135 and s136	No	Yes
Registered civil partners can be nearest relative	No	Yes, same priority as marital partners
Patient can displace nearest relative	No	Yes
Statutory right to advocacy	No	Yes
Capacitous refusal of ECT allowed for detained patients	No	Yes

The new Act has also amended the Mental Capacity Act 2005 and introduced deprivation of liberty safeguards for individuals lacking capacity. Where deprivation of someone's liberty is considered to be in their best interests, supervisory bodies (local authority for social care settings and primary care trusts for health settings) can make orders for up to 12 months to authorise deprivation of liberty, providing the person meets the eligibility criteria, which requires six assessments, including a mental capacity assessment, mental health assessment and best interests assessment.

Conclusion

GPs have an important role in caring for the mental health needs of their patients, which includes arranging or undertaking Mental Health Act assessments. GPs are often in a good position to make the second medical recommendation where they have previous knowledge of the patient. However, this may not be practicable due to busy work schedules and where patients present out of hours. Although it is not a requirement for GPs to undertake Mental Health Act assessments, it may be in the best interests of their patients to do so. Where possible patients should be encouraged to go into hospital informally before compulsion is considered.

Key points

- Mental Health Act assessments are not a compulsory requirement for GPs.
- It is generally in the interest of the patient undergoing a mental health assessment if their GP completes the second medical recommendation if the GP has prior knowledge of the patient's background.
- It is good practice to complete a joint assessment with the medical practitioner approved under section 12 (2) of the Act and the AMHP.
- GPs are most likely to be asked to undertake assessments for section 2 (admission for assessment) and section 3 (admission for treatment) but may be asked to make a recommendation for section 4, emergency admission for assessment.
- A number of new changes have been introduced by the 2007 Act, which include a change in the definition of mental disorder, changes to professional roles and the introduction of supervised community treatment. However, the process of making recommendations for compulsory detention have not changed.

Further reading and bibliography

Department of Health (2001) *The Mental Health Act. Guidance for General Practitioners: Medical Examinations and Medical Recommendations Under the Act.* DoH, London. http://www.dh.gov.uk/en/Publicationsandstatistics/Lettersandcirculars/Dearcolleagueletters/DH_4003140. Accessed 19 July 2010.

Department of Health (2008a) *Code of Practice, Mental Health Act 1983.* Stationery Office, London.

Department of Health (2008b) *Reference Guide to the Mental Health Act 1983.* Stationery Office, London.

PART 3

Treatment

CHAPTER 17

Pharmacological treatment of mental disorders

Eleni Palazidou

Case history 1

A 58-year-old man is brought to the surgery by his wife. She says he has been feeling increasingly low in mood for the last 2–3 months but did not want to see a doctor. He is miserable all the time and does not say very much. He is not interested in socialising and has been avoiding friends and family. He does not enjoy people's company any more and has stopped going to the local pub and football, activities he enjoyed in the past.

He has trouble sleeping, in particular waking up during the night and having great difficulty going back to sleep. He gets no more than 3–4 hours uninterrupted sleep. He feels tired during the day and everything has become an effort. He has to push himself to get washed and dressed for work in the mornings and has generally neglected his self-care having previously been very particular about his appearance. He is tearful and cannot see any future for himself. He feels worthless and useless and thinks his family may be better off without him. He has wished he does not wake up in the morning and has considered ending his life, but has not made any plans.

He was recently suspended from work as assistant manager of a local supermarket as he was making mistakes and his attendance had been erratic recently. He is worried that he will lose his job. He admits to drinking heavily in the last week trying to make himself feel better.

He is not known to you as they recently moved to this area so that they could be close to their daughter, who is a working single mother and needs help with childcare.

According to his previous notes he had been seen by his GP in the past complaining of anxiety and he has had periods of being unable to leave the house. He is generally an anxious person, particularly in social situations and in crowded places. He tends to avoid public transport during rush hour as he feels uncomfortable with too many people around. He has had several episodes of depression in the past and was treated with a variety of antidepressant drugs, the latest being venlafaxine, started in the psychiatric outpatients' clinic, one year ago. He felt better on this and discontinued the drug a few months ago. He has no history of mania in the past.

His mother committed suicide in her 50s when diagnosed with lung cancer, but there is no other family history of mental illness. His father had high blood pressure and died after a stroke at the age of 65. You note from his medical notes that he is a little overweight and has type 2 diabetes.

Case history 2

Stephen is in his second year of studying engineering at university. In the last month his friends and family have noticed a marked change in his behaviour. His attendance at classes is erratic and he is behind with assignments, having previously been a good student. He is isolating himself; he appears suspicious of others and gets angry for no reason. He was observed talking and laughing to himself.

At home he avoids his parents and siblings, spending his time in his bedroom chain smoking. He refuses to eat with them and prepares his own food. He has put a lot of weight on and he eats mostly junk food. The family are distressed by his behaviour, particularly as his father has recently been discharged from hospital after a heart attack and Stephen shows no interest in him. His mother is stressed out and her diabetes is out of control.

His friends persuade him to see his GP, who arranges an appointment with a psychiatrist. He tells the doctors that the voices say his parents are not his real parents; they have been replaced by imposters. He gets messages from the TV and the computer that he and his family are being used in a scientific programme initiated by NASA. He gets headaches and electric shock sensations at times, which he believes are due to them trying to remodel his brain and turn him into a robot. He says he is very scared and giggles as he says this.

Introduction

This chapter focuses on the major drug groups used in the treatment of mental disorders in primary care – antidepressants, mood stabilisers, antipsychotics and benzodiazepines. It provides practical advice on their effective use, safety and tolerability.

General principles of pharmacological treatment

Given that most drug treatments of psychiatric disorders are relatively long term, compliance is paramount. It is well established that half of the people stop or do not take their medications as prescribed. Engaging the patient in a treatment alliance is essential. Spend a little more time to explain the importance of the drug treatment and how it works and provide adequate and frank information about side-effects (see Box 17.1). This will pay dividends in the long run.

Box 17.1 Achieving therapeutic alliance

- Adequate information about the nature of their illness and the need for treatment.
- A positive message about treatability
- Dispel common myths – explain that antidepressants/antipsychotics are not addictive, do not alter one's personality nor affect the patient's intelligence
- It may take several days/weeks before they see a significant improvement in their symptoms
- They may experience some side-effects – inform them of common and serious adverse effects
- Explain that medication can be changed if they are unable to tolerate the original drug prescribed
- Regular reviewing of the patient's mental state and suicidal risk offers further reassurance and support, helps ensure compliance and allows prompt intervention in the case of any serious worsening of the condition

---

Antidepressant drugs

Case history 1

Key tasks to consider prior to commencing antidepressant drug treatment include the following:

1. Establish whether this is a depressive disorder or existential unhappiness
2. Establish whether this is unipolar or bipolar affective disorder
3. Assess suicide risk
4. Take all relevant factors into consideration before deciding on antidepressant drug choice

Action

1. The clinical picture is clearly that of depression of moderate severity and the patient is in need of antidepressant medication, although he would also benefit from concomitant cognitive behavioural therapy given his history of anxiety and the recurrent pattern of his condition (see Chapter 18).
2. Given the history of recurrent episodes of depression, and in the absence of previous manic episodes, you conclude this is a unipolar recurrent depressive disorder and you can safely start antidepressant drug treatment. A referral to the local psychiatric services is needed for advice on long-term treatment given the recurrent nature of the condition and the presence of anxiety, which worsens the outcome of depression and increases suicidal risk. If there is a history of manic episodes a psychiatric opinion should be requested urgently, as antidepressant drugs alone may trigger a manic episode and accelerate the cycle of mania/depression.
3. The risk of suicide needs to be considered when making a choice of antidepressants

Aims of antidepressant drug treatment

The ultimate aims of antidepressant drug treatment should be for the patient to return to a symptom free normal level of functioning and to stay well. In order to achieve this, the antidepressant drug treatment should be continued for a minimum of 4–6 months after full symptom control in people with a first episode of depression, in order to minimise the risk of relapse. In people who

Box 17.2 When to refer to specialist psychiatric care

- Recurrent episodes of depression
- Chronic depression
- Resistance to treatment
- High suicide risk
- Bipolar depression
- Psychotic depression

have recurrent episodes of depression, depending on their severity, duration and frequency, ongoing long-term antidepressant treatment may be required. It is advisable that a specialist opinion is sought in such cases (see Box 17.2).

Choosing the right antidepressant

The choice of antidepressant is determined by a number of factors (see Box 17.3), all of which should be taken into consideration so that the treatment is tailored to the individual to ensure compliance, efficacy and safety. The patient's concordance with the chosen drug is of primary importance (see Box 17.1).

The NICE guidelines (2009) have made antidepressant drug prescribing easier as they recommend the SSRIs as first choice antidepressants. Nevertheless, there are still some differences amongst the SSRIs themselves that may need to be taken into consideration in some patients. For example, a patient who is likely to miss occasional doses, despite advice, will be better off with a long-acting antidepressant such as fluoxetine than a short-acting one (likely to cause discontinuation symptoms) such as paroxetine. If insomnia or agitation is a key feature of the patient's presentation, then it may be advisable to avoid fluoxetine, which may exacerbate these problems. Paroxetine tends to be associated with sedation and therefore should be avoided if sedation is undesirable.

Tricyclic antidepressants tend to be used as second line antidepressants, but due to their cardiotoxic nature, they should be avoided where there is a risk of suicide, a history of arrhythmias or a recent myocardial infarction. Tricyclic antidepressants such as amitriptyline often cause sedation and are associated with troublesome side-effects such as anticholinergic effects (see Table 17.2). However, if these side-effects are particularly problematic, then nortriptyline

Box 17.3 Factors to consider in choosing the right antidepressant

- Severity of illness
- Clinical presentation
- Suicidal risk
- Previous response to treatment
- The likely tolerability of potential side-effects
- The likely benefit of potential side-effects such as sedation
- The likely drawbacks of potential side-effects such as sedation (i.e. working with machinery, driving etc.)
- Pregnancy or breastfeeding
- Concomitant treatment of physical illness or other psychiatric disorders with the potential for pharmacokinetic/pharmacodynamic interactions
- The presence of relevant physical (for example cardiovascular) disease

and lofepramine (also tricyclics) may be preferable due to their tendency to cause less sedation and fewer anticholinergic effects.

A working knowledge of all available antidepressant drug groups is needed, as many patients may have drug treatment initiated by the specialists, which may need to be continued in primary care. The evidence shows that dual action antidepressants (activating both the serotonergic and adrenergic neurotransmitter systems) such as the tricyclics, the selective serotonin and noradrenaline re-uptake inhibitors (SNRIs) and mirtazapine are more effective in more severe depression and these are more likely to be prescribed by the psychiatrists.

Mechanism of action of action of antidepressant drugs

The antidepressant drugs can be divided into three main groups on the basis of their site of action in the brain (see Box 17.4 and Table 17.1). The three main sites of action are:

1. The intraneuronal enzyme, monoamine oxidase (MAO) – the drug binds onto the MAO preventing it from breaking down the neurotransmitters noradrenaline and serotonin, which results in an increase of the concentrations available for release by the neuronal terminal into the synaptic cleft.

> # Box 17.4 Antidepressant drug groups according to site of action
>
> ## A. Monoamine oxidase inhibitors (MAOIs)
> 1. Non-selective, non-reversible MAOIs
> 2. Selective, reversible (RIMAs)
>
> ## B. Monoamine reuptake inhibitors
> 1. Non-selective noradrenaline and serotonin reuptake inhibitors (tricyclics)
> 2. Selective noradrenaline and serotonin reuptake inhibitors (SNRIs)
> 3. Selective serotonin reuptake inhibitors (SSRIs)
> 4. Selective noradrenaline reuptake inhibitors
>
> ## C. Receptor selective inhibitors and novel drugs
> 1. Non-selective alpha-2 receptor antagonists (mirtazapine)
> 2. Non-selective 5-HT2 receptor antagonists
> 3. Melatonin receptor and 5-HT2 receptor antagonist (agomelatin)

2. The re-uptake site (or transporter) on noradrenergic and serotonergic neuronal terminals – the antidepressant blocks this site, preventing the neurotransmitter from being taken back into the neuronal terminal; this results in increased concentrations of the neurotransmitter in the synaptic cleft.
3. Pre- and postsynaptic receptors on serotonergic and/or noradrenergic neurotransmitter systems in the brain.

Irrespective of the site of action, the end result of the above pharmacological actions is to increase the activity of one or both of these neurotransmitter systems (serotonergic and adrenergic). More recent evidence suggests that this increase in activity is associated with increased brain-derived neurotrophin factor (BDNF) concentrations; the latter helps to enhance neuroplasticity and the reversal of stress related reduction in new cell production in the hippocampus, a key structure in the limbic system.

Antidepressant drug side-effects

Having a good working knowledge of antidepressant drugs and their actions helps anticipate side-effects and tailor the drug to the individual (see Table 17.1). For example, sedation or weight gain may be beneficial in one patient

Table 17.1 Pharmacological actions of antidepressant drugs.

Antidepressant drug	Acute mechanism of action	Undesirable pharmacological actions
Tricyclics Amitriptyline Lofepramine etc.	5-HT and NA re-uptake inhibition	Anticholinergic; antihistaminic; alpha1 adrenoceptor blockade; direct (cardiac) membrane stabilisation
SSRIs Citalopram (Cipromil) Fluoxetine (Prozac) Fluvoxamine (Faverin) Paroxetine (Seroxat) Sertraline (Lustral) Escitalopram (Cipralex)	5-HT re-uptake inhibition	
MAOIs Phenelzine (Nardil) Isocarboxazid (Marplan) Tranylcypromine (Parnate)	Inhibition of MAO-A and MAO-B isoenzymes	Interaction with tyramine and sympathomimetic drugs Irreversible and non-selective inhibition of MAO isoenzymes
RIMAs Moclobemide (Manerix)	Reversible inhibition of MAO-A	
SNRIs Venlafaxine (Efexor) Duloxetine (Cymbalta)	5-HT and NA re-uptake inhibition	
NRIs Reboxetine (Edronax) Maprotiline (Ludiomil)	NA re-uptake inhibition	
Trazodone (Molipaxin)	5-HT2 receptor blockade and 5-HT re uptake inhibition	Other receptors
Mirtazapine (Zispin)	Alpha-2 adrenoceptor blockade 5-HT2 receptor blockade 5-HT3 receptor blockade	Antihistaminic Anticholinergic
Agomelatin (Valdoxan)	Melatonin receptor antagonist\5-HT2 receptor antagonist	

but undesirable and even detrimental in another. The wide spectrum of action of some antidepressants, such as the tricyclics and mirtazapine, render them more likely to cause side-effects (see Table 17.2), but may also afford them some beneficial effects. For example, mirtazapine causes sedation and weight gain because of its powerful antihistaminic actions but is less likely to cause sexual dysfunction than most other antidepressants because of 5-HT2 receptor

Table 17.2 Side-effects of tricyclic antidepressants.

Receptor blockade	Side-effect
Anticholinergic	Dry mouth
	Blurred vision
	Urinary hesitancy (urinary retention)
	Constipation
	Memory impairment
	Aggravation of narrow angle glaucoma
Alpha1 adrenoceptor antagonism	Orthostatic hypotension
	Cardiac effects
Direct cardiac membrane effects	Sinus tachycardia
	Conduction delay
	Arrhythmias
	Sudden death
Antihistaminic	Sedation
	Weight gain
Other side-effects	Sexual dysfunction
	Impaired cognitive and psychomotor skills
	Convulsions

blockade. Delayed ejaculation is associated with paroxetine, which may be beneficial in patients with premature ejaculation.

Although the SSRIs and SNRIs are highly selective serotonin and/or noradrenaline re-uptake inhibitors without effects on other neurotransmitter systems, they are not devoid of side-effects. These are related to an increase in 5-HT and noradrenaline neurotransmission. In the case of venlafaxine for example, and in keeping with the NICE guidelines (2009), patients need to have regular cardiovascular examinations including blood pressure monitoring and a yearly ECG. The reason is that in doses of 150 mg or above, venlafaxine has higher adrenergic activity and may cause hypertension. There is also evidence that, like the tricyclics, it may have direct cardiac effects, causing Q-T interval prolongation; hence the need for ECG monitoring and caution in prescribing for patients with suicide risk.

The side-effects of SSRIs include sexual dysfunction and anorgasmia (see Box 17.5). This is a common occurrence and often patients stop the drug for this reason. Given that sexual problems are a symptom of depression, it is essential the patient is asked during the initial assessment about any sexual problems prior to treatment to avoid confusion as to the cause.

Awareness of possible pharmacokinetic and pharmacodynamic interactions is important to avoid potential toxicity. Most psychotropic drugs are

Box 17.5 Side-effects of serotonin re-uptake inhibitors (SSRIs)

Nausea/vomiting	Sweating
Abdominal pain	Anorexia
Dry mouth	Weight loss
Constipation/diarrhoea	Nervousness/agitation
Headache	Tremor
Asthenia	Convulsions
Dizziness	Dystonic reactions
Insomnia/somnolence	Sexual dysfunction (reduced libido, anorgasmia)

metabolised in the liver by the cytochrome P450 system (mostly 2D6, which also metabolises other drugs). Some drugs may inhibit or enhance the activity of these enzymes. In patients who are on more than one medication it is essential to always check for possible interactions (consult the BNF). A pharmacodynamic interaction essential to know about as regards antidepressant drug prescribing is the risk of 'Serotonin Syndrome', a potentially lethal condition caused by excessive serotonergic activity, which is particularly likely to occur when MAOIs and SSRIs are given concomitantly.

Discontinuation syndrome

Lastly, antidepressant drugs, perhaps with the exception of fluoxetine (which has a long half-life) should not be stopped abruptly to avoid discontinuation symptoms (see Box 17.6). These are particularly troublesome when the antidepressant has a short half-life (paroxetine, venlafaxine) and can occur on withdrawal of any group of antidepressants including the tricyclics.

Indications for antidepressant drug use

Antidepressants are used not only in the treatment of depression but also in some other conditions (see Box 17.7).

Box 17.6 Antidepressant drug discontinuation syndrome

- Dizziness
- Electric shock sensations
- Anxiety/agitation
- Insomnia
- Flu-like symptoms
- Diarrhoea/abdominal spasms
- Paraesthesiae
- Mood swings
- Nausea
- Low mood

Box 17.7 Indications for antidepressant drug use other than depression

SSRIs
- Anxiety disorders
- Obsessive/compulsive disorder
- Bulimia

Tricyclics, duloxetine
- Chronic pain

Mood stabilising drugs

Patients with bipolar disorder should be seen by a psychiatrist as soon as possible, as the choice of treatment is more complex. If the patient presents in a manic state the required drug could be a mood stabiliser such as lithium, sodium valproate (epilim) or valproic acid (depakote), carbamazepine (tegretol) or lamotrigine or an antipsychotic. If there is a need for faster action, an antipsychotic would be preferable, as lithium and anticonvulsants require 5–7 days to achieve a reasonable effect.

In bipolar depressed states it is advisable to avoid antidepressants if possible because of the potential of switch into mania and/or acceleration of the bipolar cycle. Quetiapine has been shown to be effective in bipolar depression in patients with bipolar type I. It is advisable that a specialist opinion is sought prior to prescribing for bipolar depression.

Lithium

Lithium is a salt and is prescribed as lithium carbonate or lithium citrate. It is effective both in the treatment of acute mania as well as the prevention of mania, and perhaps a little less so in depressive episodes. It is also used for augmentation of antidepressants in treatment resistant depression.

Lithium has a narrow therapeutic index and its blood levels should be kept within the therapeutic range (0.6–1.00 mmol/L), not only to ensure efficacy but also to avoid toxicity. Because of its actions on the distal renal tubules, lithium is associated with increased urinary output and polydipsia. This is generally benign, but renal function needs to be monitored for the duration of the treatment to avoid renal damage. Lithium should be avoided in patients with renal disease or those in receipt of diuretics. Similarly lithium treatment can impair the production of thyroid hormone; this is not a contraindication for continuing lithium treatment, but the patient may require thyroid hormone replacement at some point in the future.

Lithium treatment is usually started in specialist care where screening tests are carried out to ensure safe prescribing and several blood levels are done over a period of a few weeks to ascertain the appropriate dose. Once a dose is established and lithium blood levels are stable, monitoring is only required at six-monthly intervals. If a patient at any time has severe gastrointestinal problems or dehydration due to other causes or develops cardiovascular or renal problems, lithium levels need to be checked and appropriate action should be taken.

Adverse effects

During lithium treatment people experience a number of symptoms which are generally well tolerated. These include mild polydipsia/polyuria, weight gain and fine hand tremor. Pretibial oedema may occur at the beginning of treatment and wears off rapidly. Some patients complain of 'emotional flatness' and slow mentation.

Long-term treatment, in addition to hypothyroidism, may in some cases cause nephrogenic diabetes insipidus, which is usually reversible on withdrawing lithium. Distal renal tubular sclerosis and glomerular morphological changes have been described. When renal damage is suspected creatinine clearance and urine and plasma osmolality (water deprivation test or 24 hour urine) should be checked.

A form of encephalopathy has been described in patients who have been concomitantly taking lithium and haloperidol long-term. Although this is an uncommon occurrence the combination is best avoided.

Toxicity

This is evident when the lithium plasma concentration is 1.6 mmol/L or above. However, even normal lithium concentrations may be associated with signs of toxicity, particularly in the elderly, and one needs to be alert to the possibility.

The early signs of toxicity are an increase in polyuria/polydipsia, coarse hand tremor and lethargy. If untreated, neurological signs, convulsions, coma and circulatory collapse can occur.

If toxicity is suspected, lithium should be immediately discontinued and blood concentrations checked as a matter of urgency, as well as urea and electrolytes. An urgent referral to the Accident and Emergency department should be made for the patient to be rehydrated and monitored. There is no antidote to lithium.

Anticonvulsants

These are mostly effective in the treatment of mania and long-term prophylaxis of bipolar disorder, with no proven efficacy in the treatment of acute depression. Lamotrigine has been shown to be effective in the prevention of depressive episodes in bipolar disorder, but its efficacy in acute mania is not established. Carbamazepine is the only drug licensed in the UK for the treatment of rapid cycling bipolar disorder (four or more episodes of mania or depression in one year). It also requires blood level measurements to avoid toxicity and it may also cause hypothyroidism.

Valproate is effective as an antimanic agent and in the long-term prophylaxis of bipolar disorder. It can uncommonly cause a fulminant hepatitis and it is advisable to do periodic liver function tests.

Pregnancy

Both lithium and anticonvulsants carry a teratogenic risk in pregnancy and ideally should be avoided. Carbamazepine is associated with spinal defects in the foetus, which may be prevented with folate supplementation during pregnancy.

It is good practice to advise patients to consider planned pregnancies and to have a discussion with a specialist about medication well in advance of conception. This is to ensure not only the avoidance of potential teratogenic effects, but also optimum monitoring and prompt and safe treatment of the illness.

Antipsychotic drugs

Introduction

Case number 2 above describes a young man with a first episode of psychosis presenting with delusions, hallucinations, passivity phenomena, inappropriate affect and impaired functioning which is most likely to be of a schizophrenic type. It is straightforward that he requires antipsychotic drug treatment. A choice needs to be made amongst the many antipsychotic drugs available. This choice will be determined not only in terms of efficacy but particularly in terms of tolerability and safety. Factors to take into consideration are the patient's age, gender, physical health (including family history of diabetes and cardiovascular disease) and other relevant factors, such as obesity.

Currently there is a range of antipsychotic drugs available, both old and new generation, and as with the antidepressants, a working knowledge of all these drugs ensures effective and safe prescribing.

The antipsychotic drugs are generally divided into two major groups: the 'first generation antipsychotics' (or 'typical') and 'second generation antipsychotics' (or 'atypical') (see Table 17.3). These categories refer to the order of

Table 17.3 Antipsychotic classes and drugs.

First generation	Second generation
Phenothiazines Chlorpromazine	**Dopamine receptor selective antagonists** Sulpiride, amisulpride, aripiprazole
Butyrophenones Haloperidol	**Dopamine and serotonin receptor antagonists** Risperidone
Thioxanthines Flupenthixol	**Wide spectrum antipsychotics** Clozapine, olanzapine, quetiapine

their appearance in the market as well as to the differences in their side-effect profile. In terms of efficacy, with the exception of clozapine, there is no superiority between one group over another. The atypical antipsychotics are a very diverse group of drugs with different pharmacological mechanisms of action, ranging from highly selective dopamine receptor antagonists to those that affect a large number of receptors within multiple neurotransmitter systems.

Side-effects

Principally, antipsychotic drugs work by blocking dopamine D2 receptors in relevant dopaminergic pathways in the brain such as the mesolimbic and mesocortical systems. Unfortunately, they (in particular the old generation antipsychotics) also affect other dopaminergic pathways such as the nigrostriatal and tuberoinfundibular pathways; these actions are responsible for their extrapyramidal side-effects and hyperprolactinaemia.

The main advantage of the second generation antipsychotics is their lower potential for extrapyramidal syndrome and hyperprolactinaemia. The extrapyramidal side-effects and in particular tardive dyskinesia are most unpleasant for the patients. Some of these are possible to counteract with anticholinergic drugs (dystonia, Parkinsonism), but others, such as akathisia or tardive dyskinesia, are difficult to treat (see Table 17.4 and Box 17.8). However, the new generation antipsychotics also have serious side-effects mostly those with a wider spectrum of action such as olanzapine, quetiapine and clozapine (see Box 17.9).

Table 17.4 Extrapyramidal side-effects (EPS) of 'first generation' antipsychotic drugs.

Type of extrapyramidal side-effect	Prevalence	Treatment
1. Parkinsonism	30%	Anticholinergic drugs Amantadine
2. Dystonia	21% (young males)	Anticholinergic drugs
3. Akathisia	25%–75%	Propranolol
4. Tardive dyskinesia	10–20% (> 1 year Rx)	Discontinue antipsychotic
5. Neuroleptic malignant syndrome	Males > females	Bromocriptine Dantrolene Diazepam

Box 17.8 Side-effects of 'first generation' antipsychotic drugs

- Extrapyramidal syndrome
- Hyperprolactinaemia: *amenorrhoea, low fertility, sexual dysfunction*
- Cardiovascular: *orthostatic hypotension, conduction delay, ventricular arrhythmias*
- Haematological
- Weight gain
- Lower seizure threshold

Box 17.9 Side-effects of wide spectrum 'atypical' antipsychotic drugs

- Weight gain
- Hyperglycaemia, insulin resistance, diabetes
- Dyslipidaemia
- Cardiovascular disease
- Fewer extrapyramidal side-effects
- Less QT prolongation
- Less hyperprolactinaemia

Patients with schizophrenia are at a higher risk of metabolic syndrome, which is a predictor of cardiovascular disease and diabetes. Three or more cardiovascular risk factors are required for a diagnosis. Drugs such as olanzapine, quetiapine and clozapine, which increase weight and raise blood sugar and lipid concentrations, increase this risk further.

In order to minimise the potential of metabolic syndrome in people on antipsychotics it is useful to monitor their weight and consider switching to another drug if weight is increasing. It is generally advisable that a weight gain of > 5% of original weight at any time during treatment is the point to do so.

Cardiac problems are not solely related to metabolic syndrome. Antipsychotic drugs, particularly some of the older ones such as haloperidol, can cause direct cardiac effects, causing conduction delays and ventricular arrhythmias leading to sudden death. Patients with known ECG abnormalities who are taking other medications with potential cardiac effects, electrolyte abnormalities etc. should be treated with great caution.

Indications for antipsychotic treatment

Antipsychotics are used primarily for the treatment of psychotic symptoms irrespective of the underlying diagnosis. They have, however, also been used occasionally as tranquillisers and this should ideally be avoided. In particular, they should not be prescribed in people with dementia, as recent evidence has shown that they increase the risk of stroke in such patients (see Chapter 12).

Antipsychotic drugs are prescribed mostly in specialist care and it is advisable always to consult a psychiatrist when initiating antipsychotic drug treatment. However, a good general understanding of how these drugs work and their potential for side-effects helps; the GP knows best the general health status of the patient and their family history and can usefully and effectively contribute in optimising treatment.

Benzodiazpines

Benzodiazepines are most commonly used in the treatment of acute anxiety and insomnia. They work by enhancing the transmission of the neurotransmitter gamma aminobutyric acid (GABA). Due to their risk of addiction and potential for withdrawal symptoms, they should be used only for a short duration (no more than a month), and where other approaches have not worked (such as relaxation and anxiety management). They should be avoided in patients with a history of substance misuse. The side-effects of benzodiazepines include headaches, blurred vision, ataxia, dysarthria and gastrointestinal problems. Paradoxical excitement may also occur. Withdrawal symptoms can occur after four weeks of use (see Box 17.10).

Insomnia

Insomnia is a common complaint and if severe can affect functioning and quality of life. Before considering the pharmacological treatment of insomnia, it is necessary to establish whether there is an underlying cause such as depression, mania, substance misuse or a physical illness, where treatment of the underlying cause may lead to resolution of the sleep problem. It is important to check that prescribed medication is being given at appropriate times such as stimulating drugs (e.g. fluoxetine) in the morning and sedating drugs in the evening (e.g. mirtazepine). Some people may also have unrealistic expectations of sleep, and the average length of sleep usually declines with age. Sleep

Box 17.10 Physical and psychological withdrawal symptoms for benzodiazepines

- Flu-like symptoms
- Visual disturbance
- Muscle weakness and paraesthesia
- Anxiety and depression
- Rebound insomnia
- Poor concentration and memory
- Delusions and perceptual abnormalities

hygiene should always be considered in the first instance, and includes simple advice such as developing a regular night-time routine (sleeping and waking at the same time), avoiding daytime naps, increasing the level of activity during the day (but not in the evening), avoiding coffee and nicotine before bedtime and only using the bed for sleeping.

Drugs used for the short-term management of insomnia are usually the short-acting benzodiazepines (e.g. temazepam) or the Z class drugs (e.g. zopiclone, zolpidem), which are structurally different from benzodiazepines but also enhance GABA transmission. NICE (2004) recommends that hypnotics are not used for more than four weeks, that the lowest therapeutic dose is used, and that the cheapest drug should be used as there is no evidence that one drug is more efficacious over another. Switching to another drug should only be considered if there is poor tolerability and should not occur due to poor response.

Key points

- It is essential to engage the patient in a therapeutic alliance in order to improve compliance with pharmacological treatment.
- The choice of antidepressant drug will depend on a number of factors including suicide risk, previous response to treatment and tolerability (and potential benefits) of side-effects.
- Both first and second generation antipsychotics are associated with serious side-effects, although 'atypicals' are less likely to be associated with extrapyramidal side-effects.
- Patients with schizophrenia are at increased risk of metabolic syndrome. Some antipsychotics (particularly 'atypicals'), such as olan-

zapine and clozapine also increase the risk of metabolic syndrome. Regular monitoring of weight and blood sugar and lipid concentration is essential.

■ Non-pharmacological approaches should be used in the treatment of insomnia in the first instance. If hypnotics are used, these should not be prescribed for more than 4 weeks and should be at the lowest effective dose.

Further reading and bibliography

Ballenger, J. C. (1999) Clinical guidelines for establishing remission in patients with depression and anxiety. *Journal of Clinical Psychology*, **60**(suppl. 22), 29–34.

Fawcett, J. and Barkin, R. L. (1997) Efficacy issues with antidepressants. *Journal of Clinical Psychology*, **58**(suppl. 6), 32–8.

Lieberman, J. A. (2005) Effectiveness of antipsychotic drugs in patients with schizophrenia. *New England Journal of Medicine*, **353**(12), 1209–23.

NICE (2009) *The Treatment and Management of Depression in Adults (update)*. Clinical guidelines CG90. National Institute for Health and Clinical Excellence, London. http://guidance.nice.org.uk/CG90.

NICE (2004) *Guidance on the Use of Zaleplon, Zolpidem and Zopiclone for the Short Term Management of Insomnia*. Technology appraisal guidance 77. National Institute for Health and Clinical Excellence, London. http://www.nice.org.uk/nicemedia/live/11530/32845/32845.pdf. Accessed 19 July 2010.

CHAPTER 18

Psychological therapies

Helen Caird, Michael Layton, Elza Tijo and Jonathan Bickford

Case history

Miss X is a 21-year-old single mother with two children: 6-year-old son M and 3-month-old daughter J.

She reported poor sleep and headaches. On assessment no organic cause was identified. Further questioning revealed her symptoms started following J's birth. She said that her sleep is disturbed partly because of waking to feed J, but she is also unable to settle once J is asleep. She is anxious about J and often feels she has to check to ensure she is lying in the correct position at night.

On direct questioning, Miss X says she is feeling low and tearful. She says that when J was first born she felt fine, as she had just moved to a newer place where she felt she could better provide for the children. Unfortunately, this meant she was further away from her parents, who had helped with childcare. The children's father had left in the months following her pregnancy with J. The pregnancy was unplanned, and when he found out he had demanded she had a termination. She had decided against this, resulting in their separation.

She has occasional suicidal thoughts, but feels protective about her children and cannot imagine them without a parental figure. She is worried that if this happens, her son will struggle as he already has behavioural difficulties at school. There were no abnormal beliefs or perceptual experiences. She had a history of depression as a teenager, when she was severely bullied at school. At that time she had some self-harming behaviour but 'has now grown out of it'.

She is keen to try psychological therapy because she does not want antidepressants while breastfeeding.

Write down your approach to this clinical scenario now and review this once you have read the chapter.

Introduction: what are psychological therapies?

Ninety per cent of people with mental health problems are cared for entirely within primary care and increasingly evidence points to the limitations of medication and the need for a range of non-pharmaceutical interventions (RCGP Curriculum, 2007). NICE guidelines promote the use of psychological therapies in the management of depression, anxiety, personality disorder and psychosis. The IAPT programme (Improving Access to Psychological Therapies) was set up to expand the workforce and psychological therapy services offered in primary care. In addition, GPs in training are required to learn about the different forms of talking therapy and may be assessed about them accordingly. So what are these therapies and how do we decide upon which patients are suitable for which type of therapy?

Psychological therapies are characterised by their interpersonal nature and so are sometimes referred to as 'talking therapies'. Psychological therapies cover both counselling and psychotherapy approaches.

Strupp (quoted in Roth and Fonagy, 2004) provides a pragmatic definition of psychotherapy:

> an interpersonal process designed to bring about modification of feelings, cognitions, attitudes, and behaviour which have proved troublesome to the person seeking help from a trained professional.

Each therapy has its own underlying model of the mind and how symptoms are to be understood. It is important to be aware of what the different therapeutic components of a therapy might be. They include: a psychological framework which allows insight into a problem, changing patterns of thought or behaviour, the experience of a non-judgemental relationship dedicated to examining the problem(s), and the opportunity to come to terms with issues such as trauma, life changes or unresolved grief. Therapy may be provided through self-help, individual sessions or in groups.

There are many competing schools of psychotherapy. This creates uncertainty which can be disheartening for some medical practitioners, who may be used to more clearly delineated pathophysiological explanations. It is helpful to remember that this uncertainty results from taking different perspectives on complex collections of potentially subjective psychological and social phenomena (such as emotions, beliefs, family networks or unconscious drives) in an attempt to generate an overarching theory of how the mind works. For the pragmatic clinician, trying to work out 'What works for whom' Roth and Fonagy (2004) provide a helpful approach for matching a patient to a type of psychotherapy.

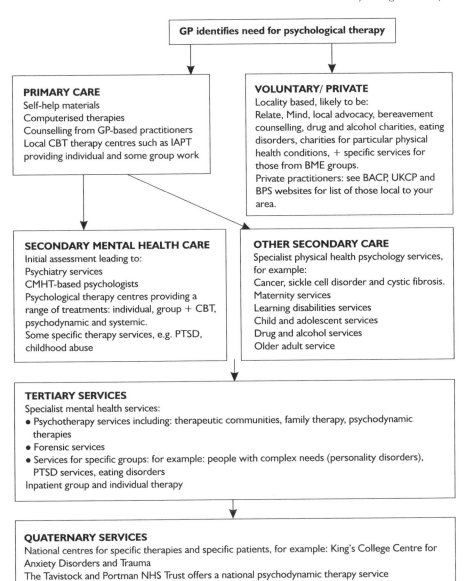

Figure 18.1 Stepped care for psychological therapies in the NHS.

Figure 18.1 gives an overview of the mainstream therapies that are available in the UK and how they fit into the NHS.

Mainstream psychological therapies

Counselling

Counselling covers a wide range of therapy styles, including Relate approaches, person-centred psychotherapy and humanistic psychotherapy. They aim to allow the patient to talk about problems in a safe and non-judgemental space, in which the therapist shows unconditional positive regard, empathy and compassion for the patient. A patient entering counselling should expect the therapist's approach to be non-directive and instead focus on listening, summarising and reflecting on the conversation. By providing the patient with an opportunity to talk about their difficulties and hear these reflected back by the therapist, counselling aims to be both a cathartic experience and to allow the patient to move forward and find their own solutions to their difficulties.

Cognitive Behavioural Therapy (CBT)

This is currently the most popular psychological therapy approach, and the one with the greatest evidence base. CBT is based on the principle that what we think can affect the way we feel and behave and that sometimes thoughts can become unhelpful to us and have a negative impact on how we feel about ourselves and the world, and thus have an impact on the way we behave. On entering CBT therapy, the therapist will explore with the patient the main problems they would like to work on and spend time uncovering the patient's unhelpful thought patterns. The therapist and patient then work together to understand the impact that such thoughts are having on how they feel and behave. The CBT approach holds that if one can learn skills to identify and then change these thought patterns, then the patient's symptoms will be relieved. The approach is strongly collaborative, with the therapist using the Socratic method of guided questioning to assist the patient to arrive at a shared formulation of the problem. The patient will be expected to take an active role in the treatment programme, often being asked to complete 'homework' between sessions. The CBT approach aims to leave the patient with a model and set of tools through which they can better understand their experiences and empower them to relieve symptoms independently of therapy.

CBT is now available as a primary care treatment as part of a stepped care model. It can be first utilised as part of an information and self-help package and then if necessary can be accessed as a one-to-one treatment through local services.

Psychodynamic/psychoanalytic therapy

Psychodynamic or psychoanalytic therapy covers a range of approaches varying in their frequency, length and intensity. Linking these approaches is their foundations in the work of Sigmund Freud and the subsequent writings of eminent psychotherapists including Anna Freud, Klein and Jung. The basic principle underlying these approaches is that the human psyche is made up of both conscious and unconscious content. Our unconscious attempts to keep difficult memories, impulses or experiences suppressed, which can result in a range of defences manifesting as symptoms, such as depression and anxiety, with which the patient presents. The aim of psychodynamic therapy is to uncover the unconscious conflicts producing a patient's symptoms. Through a patient's greater understanding of these causes, the aim is to relieve symptoms and provide the patient with a deeper and fuller insight into their psyche. A patient entering psychodynamic therapy is likely to consider childhood experiences and their effects upon their current functioning. The therapist acts almost as an interpreter for the patient's unconscious, making interpretations and linking past and present experiences on the basis of the information provided by the patient. Perhaps more so than other approaches, the therapeutic relationship between therapist and patient is central, in particular the unconscious feelings the patient may have towards the therapist. The therapist calls this the 'transference'. They interpret the transference to help understand and provide interpretations of the patient's internal conflicts.

Systemic therapy

This refers to a collection of approaches, aligned to Family Therapy, which recognise and prioritise the relationships in which a patient functions. Such approaches see patient 'problems' as residing within or between people rather than within the individual. A patient coming to systemic therapy is therefore likely to be asked to attend with their family or significant others. The focus of therapy is not on uncovering the causes of difficulties or to treat symptoms, but on understanding the meanings assigned to problems within systems and the relationship patterns that are established and maintained. By providing an opportunity for a system of people to come together to think about the ways in which they function, systemic therapy hopes to allow meanings to shift and patterns of behaviour or thinking to change. The therapist typically takes a non-expert position to facilitate discussion and highlight patterns rather than to provide the 'answer' or solution to problems.

Confidentiality

The psychotherapeutic relationship may involve a greater degree of confidentiality than most medical practitioners may be used to from fellow professionals, especially with 'information sharing' being high on the governmental and public health agenda. However, some patients require assurance of a very high level of confidentiality with a therapist, as they may wish to discuss sensitive issues such as abuse, sexuality, relationship problems or family problems. As a result, some reports from a psychotherapist may say little more than 'thank you for the referral, I have seen this patient 10 times and discharged them'. Individual practice is very variable on this issue, and may reflect the approach of the therapist as much as the wishes of the patient. The patient may well be your best guide as to the overall outcome of the therapy (Do they feel better?) without having to divulge any sensitive details. Having said this, therapists registered with a professional body or respected therapy organisation will be subject to the same rules of public interest disclosures if the patient or others are at serious risk.

Selection of patients and therapies

To match a patient to a particular therapy, it is important to consider the evidence base (and its limitations) and the relevant characteristics of that therapy as well as the patient and their circumstances.

Questions to consider include:

- What is the therapy designed to treat?
- What is the likely frequency, duration and number of sessions?
- What is the therapist's approach and focus?
- Will the patient's needs be met by this approach?
- Does the patient have a sufficient level of motivation, commitment and resilience?

Table 18.1 highlights the characteristics of each therapy. Note that these are general indicators only and the length and focus of therapy can differ widely depending upon a therapist's style and patients' needs. Some approaches may be intuitively appealing to different people. A brief description of the therapy may help someone make their decision. For example, with CBT there is an expectation of shorter term work, focusing on the present, and doing homework to try out new solutions. This may appeal to more pragmatic individuals,

Table 18.1 Summary of mainstream therapies.

Therapy	Evidence for effectiveness with	Availability	Focus	Length	Therapist
Counselling	Mild/moderate depression (NICE, 2009)	Mainly primary care	Specific problem or issue, normally focussed on present	8–10 weekly 50 minute sessions	As a minimum a certificate in counselling. May not have specialist health background
Cognitive behavioural therapy (CBT)	Mild, moderate and severe depression (NICE, 2009), anxiety, OCD (NICE, 2005), bipolar (NICE, 2006); eating disorders (NICE, 2004), schizophrenia (NICE, 2009)	Primary, secondary, tertiary and quaternary	Current thoughts and behaviours. Collaborative approach, work between sessions	From 6–12 weekly 50 minute sessions, but some flexibility	Usually health professionals with additional training
Psychodynamic	Eating disorders (NICE, 2004) Depression, anxiety (Roth and Fonagy, 2001) \ Borderline Personality Disorder (Bateman and Fonagy, 2001)	Mainly tertiary and quaternary	Longstanding difficulties, childhood, relationship to therapist	Between 1 and 2 years on NHS + some shorter term options now available	Usually health professionals with additional training
Systemic	Children and their families, people with complex networks; bipolar (NICE, 2006), eating disorders (NICE, 2004); schizophrenia (NICE, 2009)	Secondary, tertiary and quaternary	Patterns within family or system	Up to approx. 10 sessions, 60–90 minutes, fortnightly or less often	Usually health professionals with additional training

Table 18.2 Primary care psychological therapies recommended for specific diagnoses.

Diagnosis	Therapy
Mild and moderate depression	NICE (2009): guided self-help, computerised CBT, problem-solving therapy, CBT, counselling
Panic disorder	NICE (2004): CBT, self-help
Generalised anxiety disorder	NICE (2004): CBT, self-help

but some may find this intrusive or too didactic. Psychoanalytic approaches are less structured, longer term, and look at past experiences, childhood and the relationship with the therapist. They may expect the patient to talk about whatever comes into their mind and so tolerate uncomfortable thoughts and silences. Systemic approaches may be particularly useful for families or groups of carers who are struggling with someone they identify as mentally ill. Systemic approaches tend to challenge the way individuals are thought about by their network. This means that some members of the network will need to be able to attend sessions.

The other important dimension to consider when matching a patient to a therapy is the diagnosis they have received, as well as the level of risk and distress with which they present. Consequently, therapy in primary care should be aimed at individuals who do not have complex psychiatric needs. Tables 18.2 and 18.3 highlight these considerations:

Table 18.2 demonstrates the efficacy of CBT across different psychiatric diagnoses. This evidence base has been built through the wide use of Randomised Controlled Trials (RCT). It is worth noting, however, that the CBT

Table 18.3 Features which indicate the need for secondary care referral.

Referral to secondary care	Disorder
Invariably 'refer on'	Enduring severe mental illness, sexual/violent offenders, treatment-resistant mental illness
The need to 'refer on' depends on the level of complexity and risk, as well as the individual experience of the GP and therapist	Dependence on substances or alcohol, OCD, PTSD, previous therapy failure, dementia, acquired brain injury, significant risk (suicide, violence, child protection), learning disability, autism spectrum disorder, personality disorder, postnatal depression, eating disorders

approach is symptom-focused and so is better able than other approaches to demonstrate measurable change as a result of treatment. Other therapy approaches are less structured and so are less amenable to RCT research. This means that alternative approaches may be effective treatments for these diagnoses, but may not have the level of evidence needed to prove this currently.

The referring GP may also be influenced by the services and resources available locally. However, it is hoped that waiting lists and local economic pressures do not deter practitioners from identifying and offering a suitable therapy for his or her patients.

The RCGP Curriculum (2007) stresses patient-centred practice in the management of mental health problems, and evidence confirms that without it patients are less likely to commit and adhere to a management plan. Accordingly, patients should be informed of what therapies are available, and what they may expect to experience during sessions, in order to reach a decision on management together.

Those who are eligible for primary care therapies are at lower risk, so an immediate decision about treatment is often not needed. Patients and the GP can take some time to clarify issues before deciding on a management plan.

Meeting individual needs

Psychotherapy has commonly been criticised for being restricted to the well-off, educated caucasian European and American middle classes. Consideration should be given to factors in an individual's background, physical health, education and culture which may influence both the health professional's perceptions of the patient and the patient's awareness and expectations of therapy. Black and minority ethnic groups may experience a range of barriers in accessing psychological services. The gender of the therapist may be very important to some patients for many reasons (for example cultural factors or experiences of abuse). Individuals with developmental needs (children, adolescents, people with learning disability or autism) may need a specialist referral to access a modified approach, a systemic approach or the use of a creative therapy. There may be more specialised and voluntary provision in metropolitan areas.

Psychological therapies and the GP consultation

Learning is best achieved when we experience and participate in what we are trying to learn. It is likely that GPs are already using some of the skills used in psychological therapies and have ample opportunities to develop these skills further to support their patients during consultations. It has long been recognised that the interactions between GPs and patients can potentially have a therapeutic effect, for example, the role of 'doctor as drug' was noted by Balint in 1957. Practice can be informed by:

- *Counselling*
By listening to our patients, supporting and caring for them without judgement, we are acting as counsellors.

- *Cognitive behavioural therapy*
Listening out for our patient's negative thoughts may provide an opportunity within the consultation to explore their origin. For example, Socratic exploration of a depressed mother's negative comments about her inadequacy as a mother may reveal unrealistic expectations and standard setting about mothering.

- *Psychodynamic psychotherapy*
Reflecting back to the irritable patient that he seems angry with the doctor when the reasons for this cannot be identified may reveal his transference of the anger directed at himself or others. The realisation that a doctor's mood is lowered during a consultation may be a projection of a patient's lowered mood, exploration of which could lead to a diagnosis of depression.

The GP curriculum suggests that GPs have plans for how they manage their own mental health, studying and maybe trying out an online CBT course may both support this and lead to further learning of psychotherapeutic skills.

Using medication (combination treatment)

The NICE guidelines (2009) are broadly supportive of combining antidepressants with therapy, for all but mild cases of depression and anxiety. It is generally preferable to take account of individual preferences and circumstances, with an increasing need for using antidepressants where cognition and motivation are impaired. The use of benzodiazepines for anxiety disorders is generally discouraged, and is usually counterproductive if the patient is having CBT, especially for panic attacks.

Analysis of case study

Miss X has evidence of a recurrence of moderate depression which could be treated in primary care with CBT or counselling. Psychosis and significant risks have been excluded, but she warrants further monitoring by her GP. Her preference for psychological therapy is in keeping with guidelines for treatment of depression. The following factors might feature in your thinking about what to offer her:

- What therapies are available locally?
- Can she arrange childcare for the sessions?
- Her expectations of therapy (this may reflect cultural issues)
- Her level of motivation and concentration to engage with therapy
- History of bullying at school – are there underlying learning problems (past or present) which might interfere with mainstream therapy, e.g. unable to read self-help guides due to dyslexia, or a dislike of 'homework' component of CBT?
- Gender of therapist
- Possible past treatment success/failure (she has been depressed before – what treatment did she have? Was she known to CAMHS?)
- Possible childhood/personality difficulties (self-harm and personal history, and may need more exploration by GP)
- Additional practical support measures – health visitor, extended family

In the absence of complicating factors she may be suitable for counselling or CBT as a first line intervention. Complicating factors might suggest a referral on to secondary care (ideally a perinatal service), use of a longer term approach, or reconsideration of an antidepressant which is safe in breastfeeding such as sertraline.

Key points

- Psychological therapies vary in their nature and evidence base.
- They provide effective treatment for anxiety and depression in primary care.
- They require thoughtful assessment and a patient-centred approach.
- The choice of which therapy to use is guided by the complexity of the case and assessment of risk.
- A combination of antidepressant therapy and psychological therapy may be beneficial in patients with depression or anxiety disorders.

Further reading and bibliography

Bateman, A., Brown, D. and Pedder, J. (2000) *Introduction to Psychotherapy: an Out-line of Psychodynamic Principles and Practice*. Routledge, London.

Dallos, R. and Draper, R. (2006) *An Introduction to Family Therapy: Systemic Theory and Practice*. Open University Press, Berkshire.

Roth, A. and Fonagy, R. (2004) *What Works for Whom?*, 2nd edn. Guilford Press, Hove.

Simos, G. (2002) *Cognitive Behaviour Therapy: a Guide for the Practicing Clinician*. Brunner-Routledge, East Sussex.

Tudor, L. E., Keemar, K., Tudor, K., Valentine, J. and Worrall, M. (2004) *The Person-Centred Approach: a Contemporary Introduction*. Palgrave Macmillan, Basingstoke.

Index